Orthopaedics
for the
House Officer

D0555999

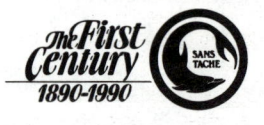

The First Century 1890-1990
SANS TACHE

Orthopaedics for the House Officer

William J. Mallon, M.D.

Michael J. McNamara, M.D.

James R. Urbaniak, M.D.

Division of Orthopaedic Surgery
Department of Surgery
Duke University Medical Center
Durham, North Carolina

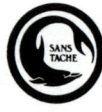

WILLIAMS & WILKINS
Baltimore • Hong Kong • London • Sydney

Editor: Michael G. Fisher
Associate Editor: Marjorie Kidd Keating
Copy Editor: Judith F. Minkove
Designer: Dan Pfisterer
Illustration Planner: Lorraine Wrzosek
Production Coordinator: Raymond E. Reter
Cover Designer: Dan Pfisterer

Copyright © 1990
Williams & Wilkins
428 East Preston Street
Baltimore, Maryland 21202, USA

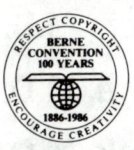

Accurate indications, adverse reactions, and dosage schedules for drugs are provided in
this book, but it is possible that they may change. The reader is urged to review the package
information data of the manufacturers of the medications mentioned.

Printed in the United States of America

Library of Congress Cataloging in Publication Data

Mallon, Bill.
  Orthopaedics for the house officer/William J. Mallon, Michael J. McNamara, James R.
Urbaniak.
    p. cm.—(The House officer series)
    Includes bibliographical references.
    ISBN 0-683-05420-1
  1. Orthopaedics.   I. McNamara, Michael J.   II. Urbaniak, James R.   III. Title.   IV. Series.
  [DNLM: 1. Emergency Medicine—methods.   2. Orthopedics—methods.   3. Wounds
and Injuries—therapy.   WE 168 M255o]
RD731.M25   1990
617.3—dc20
DNLM/DLC
for Library of Congress   89-21453
                                                                                          CIP

          90 91 92 93 94
  1 2 3 4 5 6 7 8 9 10

Preface

Orthopaedics for the House Officer is another volume in the series of introductory books intended for use by residents, interns, and medical students. It is not intended to be an encyclopaedic treatise on orthopaedic surgery. Our intention in writing this book was to produce a volume that could be carried by house officers or medical students in their lab coats for easy reference while in the emergency room or on their orthopaedic surgery rotations.

This book is designed to be used by junior residents in orthopaedics, general surgery interns and residents while on their orthopaedic or emergency room rotations, emergency room physicians, family practice physicians, physicians' assistants, and medical students.

Included herein are, hopefully, all the situations that any of the above health-care providers might encounter while in the emergency room or on the orthopaedic ward. In short, fractures and dislocations are covered in some depth, as well as the basic principles of treatment of fractures and dislocations. Cast work, splinting, traction and orthopaedic wound care are also covered in detail. Perioperative care of the orthopaedic patient is discussed in the final chapter. Elective orthopaedic procedures, such as total joint replacement, are discussed only briefly. Congenital and rheumatic diseases, which are usually seen only in the clinic setting, are also mentioned only in passing.

We gratefully acknowledge the assistance and expert advice of our publishers and editors at Williams & Wilkins. We also thank Linda Lefevre of the Duke University Medical Art Department for her production of the many excellent illustrations included in the book. For assistance in reviewing early drafts of certain chapters, our thanks are also extended to John Michael, CPO, Chief of the Division of Prosthetics and Orthotics at Duke University Medical Center and Salutario Martinez, M.D., Chief of the Divison of Skeletal Radiology, Department of Radiology, Duke University Medical Center. Finally, we are grateful to Karen Mallon, Elizabeth Justen, and Muff Urbaniak for their patience and understanding throughout the many hours the project demanded.

William J. Mallon, M.D.

Michael J. McNamara, M.D.

James R. Urbaniak, M.D.

Contents

Chapter 1

Language of Orthopaedics

Orthopaedic surgery is a diverse subspecialty that encompasses the diagnosis and treatment of abnormalities of the musculoskeletal system. These abnormalities may arise from systemic diseases (sickle cell, spondyloarthropathies), acute injuries (fractures), or idiopathic causes (idiopathic scoliosis). This book is intended to be a primary reference for the triage and treatment of common orthopaedic problems. It is not intended to be a comprehensive dissertation on musculoskeletal disease.

The most important facet of orthopaedics is the physical examination and subsequent differential diagnosis of an injury or disease state. In order to perform an accurate physical assessment, the examiner must have a working knowledge of the anatomy of the musculoskeletal system. Many injuries do not have radiologic findings, and the diagnosis is made on the basis of the clinical examination.

The structural center of the musculoskeletal system is bone. Bone gives rigidity to the musculoskeletal system. Ligaments, tendons, muscles, and nerves all function to position the skeleton in space.

Bone[2,3,4]

Bone forms by two pathways: intramembranous and endochondral ossification. The flat bones of the skeleton are formed by intramembranous ossification, in which the embryonic mesenchymal cells proliferate to form fibrous membranes where the bone is to be formed. These membrane cells directly secrete a matrix (osteoid) which can be rapidly calcified. This is termed the primary ossification center, and it is rapidly invaded by capillaries and organized into mature bone. This process of ossification proceeds outward from the primary ossification center over the entire membrane. At the completion of this embryonic growth, further bone growth occurs by the peripheral deposition of bone by the periosteum.

Endochondral ossification is the process of bone formation from a cartilage framework. This bone formation is seen in the long bones of the skeleton. Early in the embryonal state, mesenchymal cells aggregate into models of the future long bones. These cells differentiate into cartilage models, and subsequently ossify. The outside cell layer differentiates into periosteum and contributes compact bone peripherally. The calcified cartilage is degraded by chondroblasts to form what is termed the primary spongiosa, which is invaded by osteoblasts. These cells align themselves on the remaining strands of calcified cartilage, and deposit bone upon them.

Long bone elongation occurs by the expansion of the cartilage model, and primary ossification of the cartilage model until after birth. After birth, secondary growth centers appear, and develop into the epiphysis and the physeal (or growth) plate, or physis. These growth centers become the principal contributors to axial growth.

Throughout life, bone is actively turning over and remodeling. In both cortical (dense) and cancellous (spongy) bone there is active resorption and formation of bone. This rate of bone activity tends to decrease with age during adult life.

By virtue of its growth centers, bone divides itself readily into three distinct sections: the epiphysis, metaphysis, and diaphysis. (Fig. 1-1) The epiphysis lies at the end of the bone on the joint or articular side. The metaphysis is the flare of bone adjacent to the epiphysis which lies towards the shaft side of the bone. Finally the diaphysis is the shaft portion of a long bone.

Fracture Description

The appearance of the injured extremity must be carefully described in the initial evaluation of the patient. In reviewing the initial radiographs, the fracture should be accurately described. Sufficient detail must be given so that the fracture could be envisioned without the films.

The initial examination of the fracture should determine if the fracture is open or closed. The **ENTIRE** extremity must be examined for an open wound. Open fractures are classified by the grading system outlined in Table 5-1 (see Chapter Five - *Orthopaedic Emergencies and Emergency Room Techniques*).

Fractures are described systematically using the following categories: (1) location, (2) angulation, (3) amount of displacement, (4) fracture line description,

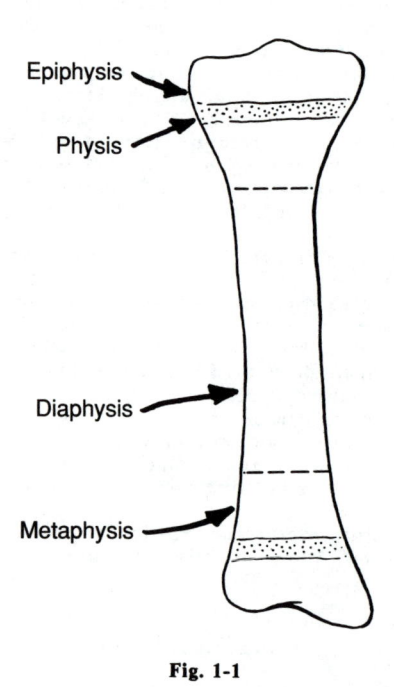

Fig. 1-1

The Four Main Parts of a Long Bone.

and (5) additional associated injuries (vascular status, compartment syndromes, dislocation).

The location of the fracture describes which bones have been fractured, and the approximate location of the fracture. In fractures of the long bones, the diaphysis is divided into thirds (i.e., proximal third, middle third, distal third). When the fracture extends into a specific area of the bone, this is included in the description (tibial plateau, intertrochanteric region of the femur). In evaluation of the initial films, a determination must be made if the fracture is entirely extraarticular, or if there is some intraarticular extension.

Fracture angulation can be described using two methods. The first method describes the relationship of the bone distal to the fracture site with respect to the proximal fragment. Using this method, a common fracture of the wrist known as a Colles' fracture would be described as a fracture of the distal radius with dorsal angulation of the distal fragment. The preferred method is to describe the apex of the fracture (Where does the fracture point?). A Colles' fracture would then be described as a fracture of the distal radius with the apex of the fracture angled volarly. In minimally displaced fractures, there is often no displacement or angulation and this description is omitted. When displacement or angulation has occurred, the fracture description should also include an estimate of the displacement or overlap. If the fractured bone ends remain in opposition, the amount of angulation can be measured in degrees. If the fractured bone ends are overriding, the amount of shortening should be measured on the radiograph.

The direction of the fracture line should always be included in the description. The fracture line or lines should be examined, and if there are more than two fragments, regardless of their size, the fracture is described as comminuted. When there appears to be a major fracture line, the direction of this through bone should be described. The direction of the fracture line corresponds to the direction and magnitude of the force applied to cause the fracture. Most commonly fractures are transverse, oblique, or spiral.

Fracture description can be difficult. The goal remains to project a mental image of the fracture to an associate who does not have the radiographs available. Beware of eponyms. From a clinical or therapeutic standpoint, it is more beneficial to describe a fracture as it viewed anatomically rather than relying on eponyms.

Further details of fracture description are discussed in Chapter Six (*Fractures, Dislocations, and Other Musculoskeletal Injuries*).

Measurements and Terms[1]

The diagnosis and treatment of musculoskeletal injuries and disease require a careful physical examination. Descriptive terms not commonly used in other medical specialties are basic vocabulary for orthopaedic surgeons, and a partial listing is included.

VARUS and VALGUS: These terms describe the angular relationship of the distal part to the proximal part around a known axis. VARUS means that the distal part is angled medially relative to the proximal part, and VALGUS (note the letter "L") means that the distal part is angled laterally.

MEDIAL and LATERAL: These terms describe the relationship to the midline, MEDIAL being closer to the midline, and LATERAL being further from the midline.

ADDUCTION and ABDUCTION: These words describe motion in the plane of the body towards (AD-duction) or away from (AB-duction) the midline. Raising the arm above the head in the plane of the shoulder requires that the shoulder be abducted. The reverse of this motion is ADDUCTION. In the distal appendicular skeleton, the terms can be more confusing. To move the great toe inward is to ABDUCT it in relationship to the normal anatomy of the foot. Therefore the abductor hallucis lies on the medial side of the foot.

PLANTAR- and DORSIFLEXION: These terms refer to the up and down motion of the ankle joint and foot. To point the toe downward, the ankle must be PLANTARFLEXED. To pull the toes and foot up, the foot is DORSIFLEXED.

SUPINATION and PRONATION: These are descriptive terms for the inward and outward rotation of the forearm and the foot. This is best remembered by the mnemonic "Pick the 'soup' up and 'pro' it away." With the hand fully supinated the palm is up; with it pronated, the palm is down. In reference to the foot, in pronation the sole (plantar surface) of the foot is turned outward, while in supination it is turned inward. In runners, pronators will run on the inside border of the shoe, and in supinators, the outside border of the shoe will show excessive wear.

RADIAL and ULNAR DEVIATION: Because the forearm bones shift their position medially or laterally with pronation and supination, the forearm bones are used to describe angulation of the hand or forearm. RADIAL or ULNAR DEVIATION implies an angulation towards the corresponding bone. This eliminates any confusion regarding medial or lateral deviation. For example, patients with rheumatoid arthritis, commonly present with an ulnar deviation or drift of the fingers.

INVERSION and EVERSION: These positions refer to the location of the forefoot in relationship to the ankle. In INVERSION, the forefoot is medial to the ankle, while in EVERSION, the forefoot is lateral to the ankle.

VOLAR- AND DORSIFLEXION: These terms refer to the motion of the wrist joint. The <u>VOLAR</u> aspect of the hand and forearm consists of the palm and the flexor surface of the forearm. The extensor surface of the forearm and hand is also known as the dorsal surface. Motion of the wrist is described as flexion toward the volar (palmar) or dorsal surfaces.

PRONE and SUPINE: These terms refer to the position of the patient on the operating or examining table. In the <u>SUPINE</u> position the patient lies on his back, and in the <u>PRONE</u> position the patient lies face-down.

CAUDAD and CEPHALAD: <u>CEPHALAD</u> refers to an orientation towards the head from a specific reference point, while <u>CAUDAD</u> refers to an orientation towards the feet from a reference point. These terms are most frequently used in the description of radiologic studies.

SAGITTAL: <u>SAGITTAL</u> describes a longitudinal plane passing through the body in an anteroposterior direction. It is most often used in CT and MR imaging to describe the orientation of the imaged slices in the study. Sagittal cuts are oriented in the long axis of the body, parallel to the midline.

CORONAL: A synonymous term is <u>FRONTAL</u>. The <u>FRONTAL or CORONAL</u> plane is a longitudinal plane passing through the body from side to side (i.e., from the left to the right or vice-versa). The <u>CORONAL</u> image is often used to describe the orientation of the study in CT or MR imaging. Coronal sections are becoming widely employed in magnetic resonance imaging, especially in orthopaedic oncology. The coronal orientation produces image slices oriented in the frontal plane of the body.

AUTOGENOUS and ALLOGENOUS: In orthopaedics many reconstructive procedures require bone grafts. When the graft is taken from the same host, it is referred to as an <u>AUTOGENOUS</u> graft. When bone from another host is used it is referred to as an <u>ALLOGENOUS</u> graft, or <u>ALLOGRAFT</u>. In rare instances, a graft from another species can be used, and these are known as xenografts.

IPSILATERAL and CONTRALATERAL: These terms describe the orientation with respect to a fixed point. <u>IPSILATERAL</u> refers to the same side as the orientation point, while <u>CONTRALATERAL</u> refers to the side away from the reference point.

Common Orthopaedic Abbreviations

AbPB	-	abductor pollicis brevis
AbPL	-	abductor pollicis longus
ACL	-	anterior cruciate ligament
AdP	-	adductor pollicis
AFO	-	ankle-foot orthosis
AO	-	Arbeitsgemeinschaft fuer Osteosynthesfragen. This is a Swiss-based group that studies internal fixation of fractures.
AROM	-	active range of motion
ASIF	-	Association for the Study of Internal Fixation. This is the American counterpart of the AO group.
CDH	-	congenital dislocation of the hip
CORR	-	*Clinical Orthopaedics and Related Research*
CPM	-	continuous passive motion
CTLS	-	cervico-thoraco-lumbo-sacral (as in CTLS brace)
CTS	-	carpal tunnel syndrome
DIP	-	distal interphalangeal joint
DIPJ	-	distal interphalangeal joint
ECRB	-	extensor carpi radialis brevis
ECRL	-	extensor carpi radialis longus
ECU	-	extensor carpi ulnaris
EDC	-	extensor digitorum communis
EDQ	-	extensor digitorum quinti
EHL	-	extensor hallucis longus
EIP	-	extensor indicis proprius
EPB	-	extensor pollicis brevis
EPL	-	extensor pollicis longus
ESR	-	erythrocyte sedimentation rate
EWHO	-	elbow-wrist-hand orthosis
FCR	-	flexor carpi radialis
FCU	-	flexor carpi ulnaris
FDP	-	flexor digitorum profundus
FDS	-	flexor digitorum superficialis
FHL	-	flexor hallucis longus
FPB	-	flexor pollicis brevis
FPL	-	flexor pollicis longus
FOB	-	foot of bed (as in "Elevate FOB")
FROM	-	full range of motion
FWB	-	full weightbearing
F_x	-	fracture
HKAFO	-	hip-knee-ankle-foot orthosis
HNP	-	herniated nucleus pulposus

HOB	-	head of bed (as in "Elevate HOB")
HTO	-	high tibial osteotomy
ITB	-	iliotibial band
JBJS	-	*Journal of Bone and Joint Surgery*
JHS	-	*Journal of Hand Surgery*
JPO	-	*Journal of Pediatric Orthopaedics*
KAFO	-	knee-ankle-foot orthosis
LAC	-	long-arm cast
LLC	-	long-leg cast
LROM	-	limited range of motion
L/S	-	lumbosacral (as in L/S corset)
MCL	-	medial collateral ligament
MCP	-	metacarpophalangeal joint
MCPJ	-	metacarpophalangeal joint
MTP	-	metatarsophalangeal joint
MTPJ	-	metatarsophalangeal joint
NHP	-	nursing home placement
N/V	-	neurovascular
ORIF	-	open reduction and internal fixation
PCL	-	posterior cruciate ligament
PFFD	-	proximal femoral focal deficiency
PIP	-	proximal interphalangeal joint
PIPJ	-	proximal interphalangeal joint
PROM	-	passive range of motion
PT	-	physical therapy
PT	-	pronator teres
PTB	-	patellar-tendon bearing
PWB	-	partial weightbearing
ROM	-	range of motion
SAC	-	short-arm cast
SLC	-	short-leg cast
STS	-	soft-tissue swelling
TAM	-	total active motion
TDWB	-	touchdown (or toe down) weightbearing
THA	-	total hip arthroplasty
THR	-	total hip replacement
TJA	-	total joint arthroplasty
TJR	-	total joint replacement
TKA	-	total knee arthroplasty
TKR	-	total knee replacement
TLS	-	thoraco-lumbo-sacral (as in TLS corset)
TPM	-	total passive motion
TSR	-	total shoulder replacement
TT	-	tourniquet time
TTT	-	total tourniquet time
VSS	-	vital signs stable
WBAT	-	weightbearing as tolerated
WHO	-	wrist-hand orthosis

References

1. Hoppenfeld S. *Physical Examination of the Spine and Extremities.* Norwalk: Appleton-Century-Crofts, 1976.
2. Lovell WW, Winter RB. *Pediatric Orthopaedics.* 2nd edition. Philadelphia: J. B. Lippincott, 1986.
3. Rockwood CA Jr, Green DP. *Fractures in Adults (Volume 1).* Philadelphia: J. B. Lippincott, 1984.
4. Rockwood CA Jr, Wilkins KE, King RE. *Fractures in Children (Volume 3).* Philadelphia: J. B. Lippincott, 1984.

Chapter 2

Orthopaedic Literature

As in all branches of medicine and surgery, an extensive literature exists in orthopaedic surgery. While younger residents are not expected to have read all of the literature, it is extremely important to know where to find some vital pieces of information.

Listed below are the books that are most commonly used by orthopaedic surgeons as references. An effort has been made in all cases to choose a more current book, where possible. Obviously, we could not include all sources and the following list should serve only as a starting point. The list is annotated to help students find sources that may be most helpful for a specific problem. At the end of the list of books, the primary journals used by orthopaedists are listed.

General Books

Campbell's Operative Orthopaedics. 7th Edition. 4 vols. AH Crenshaw, ed. St. Louis: C. V. Mosby, 1987. The so-called "bible" of orthopaedics, this is still the standard reference although it has been challenged recently by Evarts' and Chapman's texts (next selections). It is mostly an operative technique book and is not a good source for closed fracture treatment.

Surgery of the Musculoskeletal System. 4 vols. CMcC Evarts, ed. Philadelphia: Churchill-Livingstone, 1983. Evarts' book is an attempt to combine the operative technique of Campbell's while including more information on nonoperative treatment of orthopaedic problems. It can be used for closed fracture treatment but rarely is in acute situations. It contains no information on pediatric orthopaedic problems.

Operative Orthopaedics. MW Chapman, ed. Philadelphia: J. B. Lippincott, 1988. Chapman's text is the newest large text on orthopaedics. Its strengths are its focus on preoperative planning for surgical problems.

Fractures (In Adults and In Children). 3 vols. CA Rockwood, DP Green, eds. (Vols. 1-2 - Adults), 2nd edition. CA Rockwood, KE Wilkins, RE King, eds. (Vol. 3 - Children), 1st edition. Philadelphia: J. B. Lippincott, 1984. This is the standard reference on fractures. The first two volumes are a revised edition and include information on both closed and open treatment of fractures. All volumes also includes sections on dislocations and ligament injuries.

Orthopaedics: Principles and Their Applications. 4th edition. 2 vols. SL Turek. Philadelphia: J. B. Lippincott, 1984. This book is often used as a single reference by medical students who find Campbell's and Evarts' too encyclopaedic. It is still quite inclusive.

Surgical Exposures in Orthopaedics. S Hoppenfeld, P de Boer. Philadelphia: J. B. Lippincott, 1984. This is a relatively new book which is a superb reference on the anatomy of virtually all orthopaedic approaches.

Physical Examination of the Spine and Extremities. S Hoppenfeld. New York: Appleton-Century-Crofts, 1976. Hoppenfeld's book on the orthopaedic physical examination should be read by all orthopaedic residents and medical students interested in orthopaedics.

Surgical Anatomy for Surgeons: The Limbs and Extremities. 3rd edition. WH Hollinshead. New York: Harper & Row, 1984. Hollinshead's book is an encyclopaedic coverage of orthopaedic anatomy. It is less clinically oriented than Hoppenfeld's book on exposures but is an excellent reference.

Books on Specific Topics - Regional

Operative Hand Surgery. 2nd edition. 3 vols. DP Green, ed. New York: Churchill-Livingstone, 1988. This is the standard reference on hand surgery. Multiple books on hand surgery are available and some may find this book a bit encyclopaedic.

The Hand: Diagnosis and Indications. 2nd edition. G Lister. New York: Churchill-Livingstone, 1984. Lister's book is a good reference for those who desire a quicker read on the basic principles of hand problems than Green's book offers.

The Wrist. J Taleisnik. New York: Churchill-Livingstone, 1985. Similar to Morrey's elbow book, Taleisnik's work is new but has quickly become the definitive text on wrist problems.

The Elbow and Its Disorders. BF Morrey, ed. Philadelphia: W. B. Saunders, 1985. This book is almost without peer among books discussing the problems of a single joint. It is highly recommended.

Surgery of the Shoulder. 3rd edition. AF DePalma, ed. Philadelphia: J. B. Lippincott, 1983. DePalma's text is a good book on shoulder surgery which has, in the past, been the standard text. It is now slightly dated and may be supplanted by Rowe's book.

The Shoulder. CR Rowe, ed. New York: Churchill-Livingstone, 1988. This recently released book is written by one of the acknowledged experts on shoulder surgery and will likely become a standard reference. The only drawback is that all the chapters are written by surgeons from one hospital, rather than from experts chosen from various centers.

The Cervical Spine. The Cervical Spine Research Society. 2nd edition. Philadelphia: J. B. Lippincott, 1989. Recently updated, *The Cervical Spine* is an excellent review with chapters written by most of the authorities on cervical spine problems.

The Spine. 2 vols. RH Rothman, FA Simeone, eds. Philadelphia: W. B. Saunders, 1982. This book discusses mostly acute trauma and adult chronic pain syndromes.

Low Back Pain: Assessment and Management. DM Spengler. New York: Grune & Stratton, 1982. Written by a physician who has published extensively on this topic, this book is a short, very readable reference.

Pelvic and Acetabular Fractures. DC Mears, HE Rubash. Thorofare, NJ: Slack, 1986. One of the two main books on a complex topic, this is the longer and more difficult book of the two. It is, however, comprehensive.

Fractures of the Pelvis and Acetabulum. M Tile. Baltimore: Williams & Wilkins, 1984. A shorter version than Mears and Rubash's book, this book clearly and adequately covers the topic.

Surgery of the Hip Joint. 2nd edition. 2 vols. RG Tronzo, ed. New York: Springer-Verlag, 1984 (Vol. 1), 1987 (Vol. 2). Tronzo's book discusses adult hip problems, including fractures, osteotomies, and arthroplasty.

Advanced Concepts in Total Hip Arthroplasty. WH Harris, ed. Thorofare, NJ: Slack, 1985. Total joint arthroplasty is a field in such flux that it is difficult for any book to be current. This book is actually a collection of papers on current concepts in this field and may be too much for someone desiring only an introduction. As an introduction, the sections in either *Campbell's Operative Orthopaedics* or Chapman's *Operative Orthopaedics* (see above) are probably the best choices.

Surgery of the Knee. JN Insall. New York: Churchill-Livingstone, 1984. Insall's book is the standard reference on the knee and covers ligamentous injuries, arthroplasty, and fractures.

Total Knee Arthroplasty: A Comprehensive Approach. DS Hungerford, KA Krackow, RV Kenna, eds. Baltimore: Williams & Wilkins, 1984. As with most books on total hip replacement, this book may be more than early students desire, but it is quite good.

Arthroscopic Surgery. 2 vols. LL Johnson. St. Louis: C. V. Mosby, 1986. This is a mammoth book with thousands of color photographs of arthroscopic procedures. It is quite comprehensive but very readable.

The Crucial Ligaments. JA Feagin Jr, ed. New York: Churchill-Livingstone, 1988. Feagin's book is the most current and popular treatise on the subject of injuries to the cruciate and collateral ligaments of the knee. It is well done, and the opening section, which presents multiple case studies of knee ligament injuries, is especially good.

Disorders of the Ankle. H Kelikian, AS Kelikian. Philadelphia: W. B. Saunders, 1985. A comprehensive review of ankle fractures and ligament problems; however, total ankle replacement is not discussed.

Disorders of the Foot. 2 vols. MH Jahss, ed. Philadelphia: W. B. Saunders, 1982. This is a very comprehensive book on all aspects of foot problems.

Surgery of the Foot. 5th edition. RA Mann, ed. St. Louis: C. V. Mosby, 1986. Mann's book is an excellent monograph which clearly covers all foot problems.

Books on Specific Topics - Pediatrics

Pediatric Orthopaedics. 2nd edition. 2 vols. WW Lovell, RB Winter, eds. Philadelphia: J. B. Lippincott, 1986. Lovell and Winter published a very readable book for their first edition but it was not as comprehensive as Tachdjian's book, which has been preferred by many pediatric orthopaedists. The second edition is a definite improvement with the revision of many of the chapters. Because it is contemporary it serves as an excellent reference on pediatric orthopaedics. Fractures, however, are not covered.

Pediatric Orthopaedics. MO Tachdjian, ed. Philadelphia: W. B. Saunders, 1972. Formerly the standard reference on children's orthopaedic problems, Tachdjian's book is now slightly dated. However, a second edition is expected to be published in early 1990. Fractures are well covered in the 1972 edition.

Skeletal Injury in the Child. JA Ogden. Philadelphia: Lea & Febiger, 1982. This is an excellent book on children's fractures by one of the top experts in the field. However, it is not used as often as Vol. 3 of *Fractures* (Rockwood, Wilkins, King).

Scoliosis and Other Spinal Deformities. 2nd edition. DS Bradford, JH Moe, JW Ogilvie, JE Lonstein, RB Winter, eds. Philadelphia: W. B. Saunders, 1987. Written by the definitive experts in this field, this book is as complete and well-written as any text in orthopaedics.

Congenital Dislocation of the Hip. MO Tachdjian, ed. New York: Churchill-Livingstone, 1982. See next reference.

The Child's Foot. MO Tachdjian, ed. Philadelphia: W. B. Saunders, 1985. Tachdjian is an acknowledged authority in pediatric orthopaedics, and both his hip and foot books are superbly done.

Clubfoot. VJ Turco. New York: Churchill-Livingstone, 1981. Turco's book is a short treatise on a difficult problem.

Complex Deformities of the Foot in Children. SS Coleman. Philadelphia: Lea & Febiger, 1983. Coleman's book is much shorter than Tachdjian's, and very readable. It includes clubfoot problems and several other difficult pediatric foot deformities.

Books on Specific Topics - Special Topics

Orthopaedic Biomechanics. VH Frankel, AH Burstein. Philadelphia: Lea & Febiger, 1970. Though an older book, this book is still quite a good introduction to biomechanics and can be read quite easily.

Manual of Internal Fixation. ME Mueller, M Allgoewer, R Schneider, H Willenegger. Berlin: Springer-Verlag, 1979. Written by the Swiss-based AO/ASIF group (Arbeitsgemeinschaft fuer Osteosynthesfragen - Association for the Study of Internal Fixation), this is the standard reference on open treatment of fractures.

External Skeletal Fixation. DC Mears. Baltimore: Williams & Wilkins, 1983. Mears' book is a comprehensive coverage of this technique. However, individual sections are not overly long and can be read easily in preparation for specific problems.

Musculoskeletal Tumor Surgery. 2 vols. WF Enneking. New York: Churchill-Livingstone, 1983. *Musculoskeletal Tumor Surgery* is a very large work covering all aspects of orthopaedic tumors - diagnosis, radiology, pathology, and treatment.

Principles of Musculoskeletal Pathology. 2nd edition. WF Enneking. Gainesville: Storter, 1981. This is a short monograph which is an excellent reference for students. Pathology is covered well but there is little on treatment.

Bone Tumors. 4th edition. DC Dahlin, KK Unni. Champaign, IL: CC Thomas, 1986. Dahlin's book has been the standard work on orthopaedic tumor pathology. It is quite good in that regard but there is little mention of treatment.

Textbook of Rheumatology. 2nd edition. 2 vols. WN Kelley, ED Harris Jr, S Ruddy, CB Sledge. Philadelphia: W. B. Saunders, 1985. This is an excellent textbook on arthritic disorders. Kelley, Harris and Ruddy are rheumatologists while Sledge is an orthopaedist. Because of the multi-disciplinary approach, both medical and surgical treatment of arthritic problems are discussed.

Diagnosis of Bone and Joint Disorders. 3 vols. D Resnick, G Niwayama. Philadelphia: W. B. Saunders, 1981. A true magnum opus, this huge, well-illustrated work comprehensively reviews radiology and pathology of arthritides and neoplasms.

Journals

Journal of Bone and Joint Surgery - American Edition (JBJS-A). If you decide to subscribe to an orthopaedic journal, this is the one with which to start. This essential journal is the most highly quoted and best refereed journal in orthopaedics. Published ten times per year.

Journal of Bone and Joint Surgery - British Edition (JBJS-B). The British edition of JBJS is predominately comprised of articles from Great Britain but also includes papers from other English-speaking countries. Published five times per year.

Clinical Orthopaedics and Related Research. Among American journals, this is probably the second most quoted reference after JBJS-A. Published monthly.

Acta Orthopaedica Scandanavica. This is an excellent journal based in Denmark and covering mostly Scandanavian orthopaedics, but written in English. It is published six times per year with two or three supplements per year which discuss a single problem.

Journal of Hand Surgery. Now available in both an American and British edition, similar to JBJS, the American edition is a must in the field of hand surgery. It is published nine times per year. The British Journal of Hand Surgery has replaced Hand, which was the former British hand journal. It is currently published five times per year.

American Journal of Knee Surgery.

American Journal of Sports Medicine.

Arthroscopy.

Journal of Arthroplasty.

Journal of Pediatric Orthopaedics.

Journal of Orthopaedic Trauma.

Journal of Spinal Disorders.

Foot and Ankle.

Spine. The above nine journals provide very good coverage of their specific sub-specialties. General orthopaedists, residents, and students rarely subscribe to these but they are often used as references.

Orthopaedics.

Contemporary Orthopaedics.

Orthopaedic Review.

Surgical Rounds in Orthopaedics.

Journal of Musculo-Skeletal Medicine.

The Physician and Sports Medicine. The above six journals are less rigidly refereed and are not as widely read by orthopaedists as the earlier journals. Students may occasionally find some interesting articles in them. Notably, Orthopaedics often carries excellent review articles, and Contemporary Orthopaedics always has a monthly panel discussion which covers one topic in depth.

Chapter 3

History and Physical Examination of the Orthopaedic Patient

The Orthopaedic History[1]

A thorough history is an integral part of the diagnosis of musculoskeletal injuries. The breadth and depth of the history should be dictated by the chief complaint. Musculoskeletal injuries can often be presenting symptoms of widespread disease processes.

Because the orthopaedic surgeon must frequently provide information about the injured patient to insurance carriers, employers, vocational rehabilitation counselors, and attorneys, specific details about the injury should be obtained and recorded, especially in work-related injuries. This information should include the following: date and exact mechanism of injury, time out of work, previous treatment and by whom, and referring physician or agency.

Acute Injury: The history of the acute injury should focus on the mechanism of the injury. The patient should be questioned about his injury. Specific questions should be addressed towards body position when the injury occurred. An assessment of the force causing the injury should be made. For example, did the patient sustain the pelvic fracture in a fall in the bathroom or a motor vehicle accident? Is the onset of pain and limitation of range of motion immediate or gradual? A classic example of the gradual limitation of motion is the nondisplaced fracture of the radial head where the patient presents to the emergency room with increasing pain and limitation of range of motion several hours after injury. When the injury occurred was there a sense of "giving way"?

Did the patient hear or feel a "click" or a "pop"? If the patient has diminished or loss of sensibility or motor power, the onset of the neurologic change, i.e., immediate or gradual, must be obtained and documented. Additional questions should focus on the patient's activities since the injury. Did the patient continue to participate in the game? Was the patient able to walk on an injured lower extremity after injury? Also, if the patient presents to the clinic some time after the injury, an effort should be undertaken to determine what are the patient's expectations and what were the reasons for delay in presentation.

Chronic Injury: Chronic injuries often require more extensive history taking. The pertinent history is often hidden in a maze of unrelated events. Many patients will unknowingly confuse dates and details. One effective means to sort out the details is to have two separate observers take the history, and then to compare the details. The radiology film jacket will often help to put dates on previous trauma or visits to the clinic if old records are unavailable.

In nonacute injuries, the time frame should first be determined. When did the injury first occur? Have there been successive flares or episodes of reinjuries? What diagnostic and surgical procedures have been performed and what were the short- and long-term results? Has the presenting disability changed in character over time? As the history taking progresses, often the open-ended question must be abandoned for more specific, detailed questions.

Constitutional symptoms should not be neglected. Questions should address signs and symptoms such as fever, chills, nausea, or vomiting. In all patients presenting to the emergency room who may require surgery, a full review of systems should be sought with emphasis on cardiopulmonary conditions that would increase anaesthetic risk.

Trauma: The orthopaedic history of the trauma patient focuses directly on the mechanism of injury. How much energy caused the injury? Are any other systems damaged? What injuries demand immediate surgical intervention and with what priority? What is the cardiopulmonary status of the patient? What are the risks of emergency anaesthesia? What is the tetanus status of the patient? Is the patient hemodynamically stable enough to permit a full evaluation in the emergency room?

Pain: Pain is a difficult symptom to describe or quantitate. The best description of the patient's pain should be detailed. The radiation of pain should be determined. Also ask the patient which movements and positions make him/her more comfortable and which make him worse.

The Physical Examination

The physical examination should begin in the examining room with the involved extremity well exposed for examination. An examination of the upper extremity requires that the entire forequarter be accessible and the patient should be draped to maintain modesty. The lumbar spine cannot be examined without the patient in a hospital gown. Categorically, an unconscious trauma patient should be entirely undressed so that occult injury is not overlooked.

The optimum examining room places the examining table in the center of the room so that the patient can be approached from either side of the table with the patient either prone or supine.

The patient should be asked to demonstrate where the pain is most severe and the motions which aggravate or relieve the condition. Many patients will not localize their pain well, and in acute trauma, it is important to ask the patient to use the <u>one finger-one spot</u> rule to localize the point of maximum pain. The injured area should be examined for atrophy or asymmetry. Other observations should include abnormal posture, and the resting or "comfortable position."

After observation of the patient, the examiner should approach the patient and begin to palpate the area of interest. A useful technique is to progress from relatively pain-free areas to the most tender or sensitive regions. Any painful maneuvers should be avoided until the end of the examination (e.g., the straight leg raise in a suspected herniated nucleus pulposus). The examination should include a minimum of a joint above and below the injury.

In chronic diseases such as rheumatoid arthritis, an extensive evaluation of all joints may be necessary to follow the progression of the disease. Observations should include assessment of inflammation, extent of synovitis, warmth and an accurate measurement of range of motion - both active and passive.

Range of Motion:[1,9] Examination of the range of motion (ROM) of the injured extremity often yields a wealth of diagnostic data as well as qualitative measurement for future examinations. Normal values for range of motion of most joints are shown in Figs. 3-1 to 3-7. The goniometer should be used to measure range of motion. An accurate range of motion assessment should include both active and passive ROM. When the the active range of motion is limited by pain this should be noted. Again, the exam should include a joint above and below the injury.

Motor Testing:[1,9,10] Examination of specific muscles or muscle groups will often give major diagnostic information to an injury or disease. Muscle strength is scored on a system of 0-5; five signifying normal strength while zero indicates no muscle activity as shown in Table 3-1. Some examiners add a plus or minus to the grading system to denote more subtle differences in motor deficits. Normal motor strength is a somewhat enigmatic term - normal motor strength in an 88-

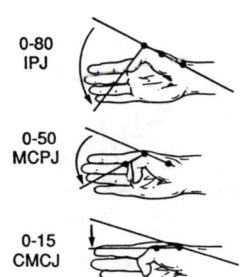

0-80
IPJ

0-50
MCPJ

0-15
CMCJ

Thumb

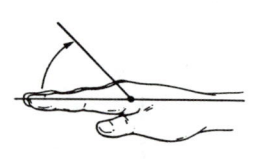

Thumb Opposition

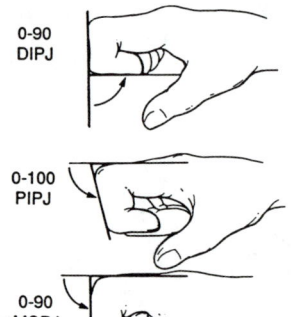

0-90
DIPJ

0-100
PIPJ

0-90
MCPJ

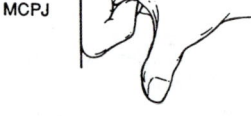

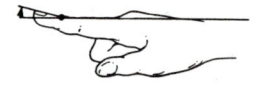

Finger Hyperextension

Fingers

Fig. 3-1

Normal Ranges of Motion for the Thumb and Fingers

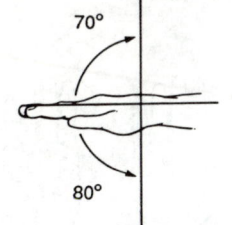

70°

80°

Wrist

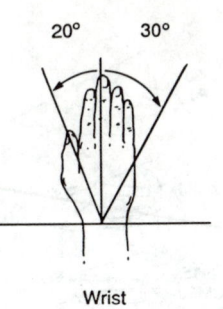

20°   30°

Wrist

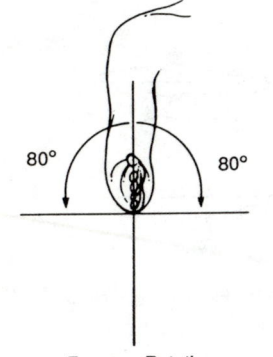

80°   80°

Forearm Rotation

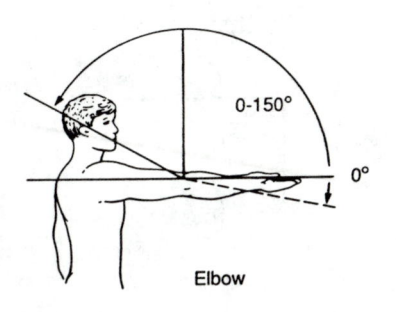

0-150°

0°

Elbow

Fig. 3-2

Normal Ranges of Motion for the Wrist and Elbow

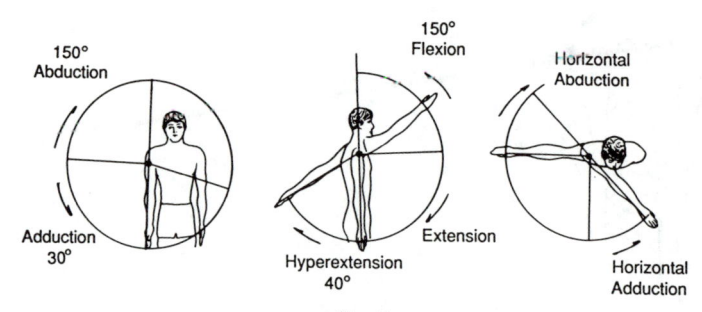

Shoulder

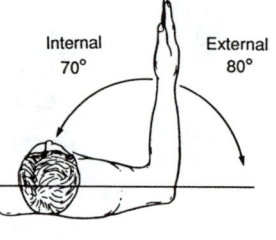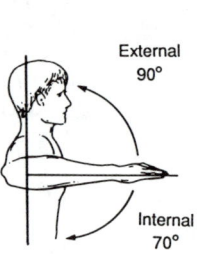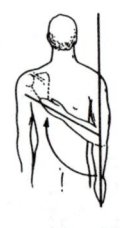

Shoulder Rotation

Internal Rotation

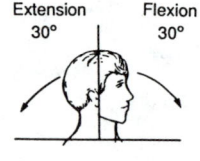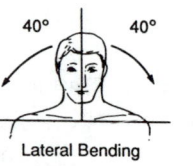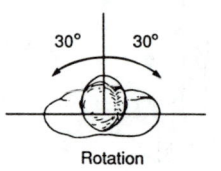

C-Spine

Fig. 3-3

Normal Ranges of Motion for the Shoulder and Cervical Spine

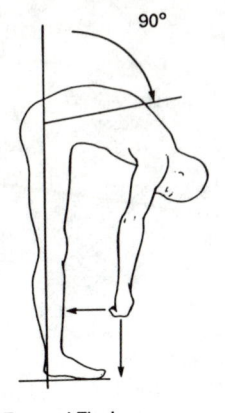

Forward Flexion

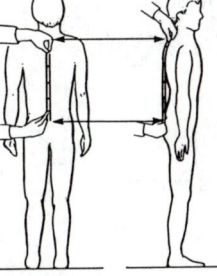

Distraction in Flexion
10 cm.

Thoraco-Lumbar Spine

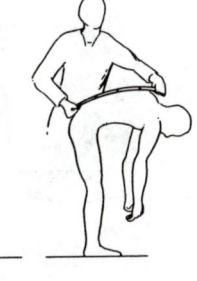

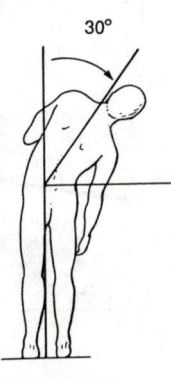

Lateral Bending

Fig. 3-4

Normal Range of Motion for the Thoracolumbar Spine

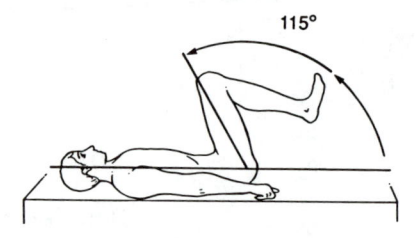

Hip Flexion

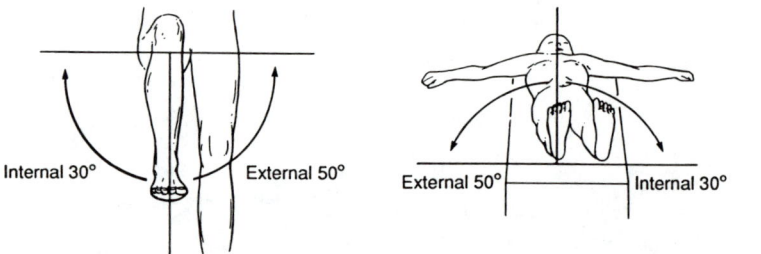

Hip Rotation in Flexion   Hip Rotation in Extension

Fig. 3-5

Normal Ranges of Motion for the Hip

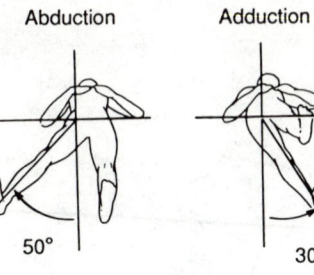

Abduction   Adduction

50°   30°

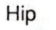

Hip

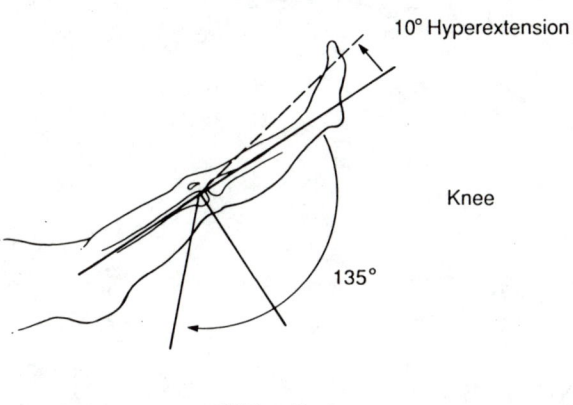

10° Hyperextension

Knee

135°

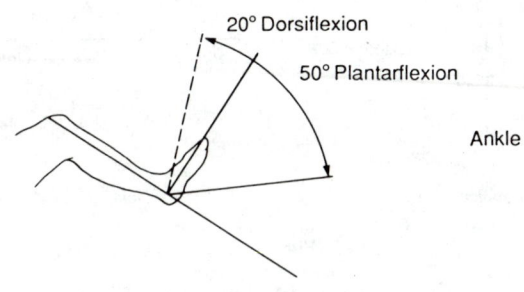

20° Dorsiflexion

50° Plantarflexion

Ankle

Fig. 3-6

Normal Ranges of Motion for the Hip, Knee, and Ankle

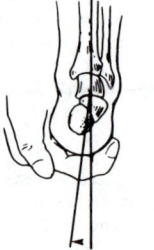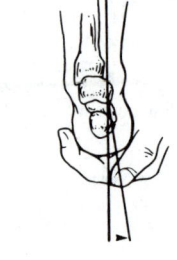

Subtalar Motion

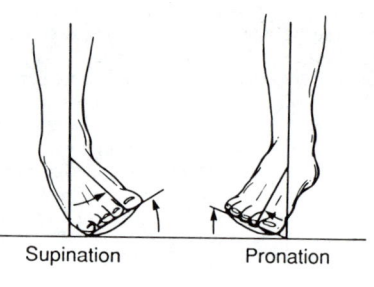

Supination   Pronation

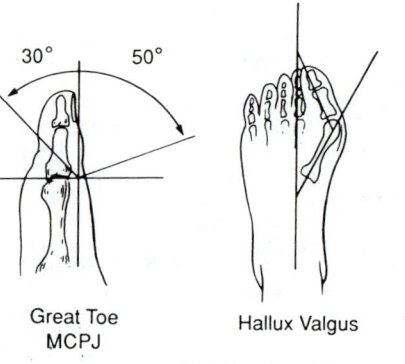

30°   50°

Great Toe
MCPJ

Hallux Valgus

Fig. 3-7

Normal Ranges of Motion for the Foot and Toes

year-old female is not normal motor strength in a professional athlete. An extremely helpful method of comparison is to measure the unaffected contralateral limb or muscle group to get a quantitative assessment of the normal. The motor exam will often give information about nerve root and peripheral nerve lesions. Although large muscle groups are innervated by contributions from several nerve roots, usually a single nerve root predominates. Tables 3-2 and 3-3 list the muscles and their innervation both by spinal root and peripheral nerves.

Reflexes:[1,9,10] No neurologic assessment is complete without deep tendon reflex testing. Reflex testing should be performed with the patient seated comfortably on the examining table with the feet off the ground. The primary reflexes are listed in Tables 3-4 and 3-5. The posterior tibialis reflex is included, although this reflex is difficult to demonstrate. The posterior tibialis reflex can be considered significant when it is present unilaterally.

In the patient with a suspected spinal cord injury, additional reflexes, especially the cremasteric and the bulbocavernosus reflexes should be tested. The bulbocavernosus reflex or its absence defines spinal shock.

The bulbocavernous reflex is tested by performing a rectal exam and, with the examining digit within the rectal vault, tugging on the glans penis, the clitoris, or an indwelling Foley catheter. An intact bulbocavernous reflex exists when the anal sphincter contracts on the examining digit.

The return of the bulbocavernosus reflex after a significant spinal injury signifies the end of spinal shock. If the patient has had absolutely no return of neurologic function below the injury level at the end of spinal shock, the prognosis for neurologic improvement is almost zero.

Sensory Testing:[1,9,10] Sensory testing should include a dermatomal examination for pin-prick and soft touch. Dermatomes are shown in Figs. 3-8 and 3-9. For this purpose, the house officer should have a ready supply of safety pins which should be discarded after each use. In addition, the patient should be asked to perform sharp - dull discrimination in areas of question. Care should be taken to delineate an insensate area to determine whether it is dermatomal in pattern. This can be particularly difficult in patients with peripheral neuropathy secondary to diabetes, vascular insufficiency, heavy metal poisoning, or leprosy (Hansen's disease). A knowledge of the autogenous zones where there is no dermatomal overlap can be helpful in the examination.

Proprioception proceeds through different spinal tracts and should be tested separately. Proprioception is assessed by requesting the patient to acknowledge the position of the extremity without vision. Grasp the toe or finger on either side rather than on the plantar and dorsal surface to eliminate pressure sensation.

In hand injuries, two-point discrimination allows for rapid and reproducible assessment of digital nerve function.[2,3,12] Two-point discrimination can be tested using blunted calipers or a paper clip bent into a "U." The patient's

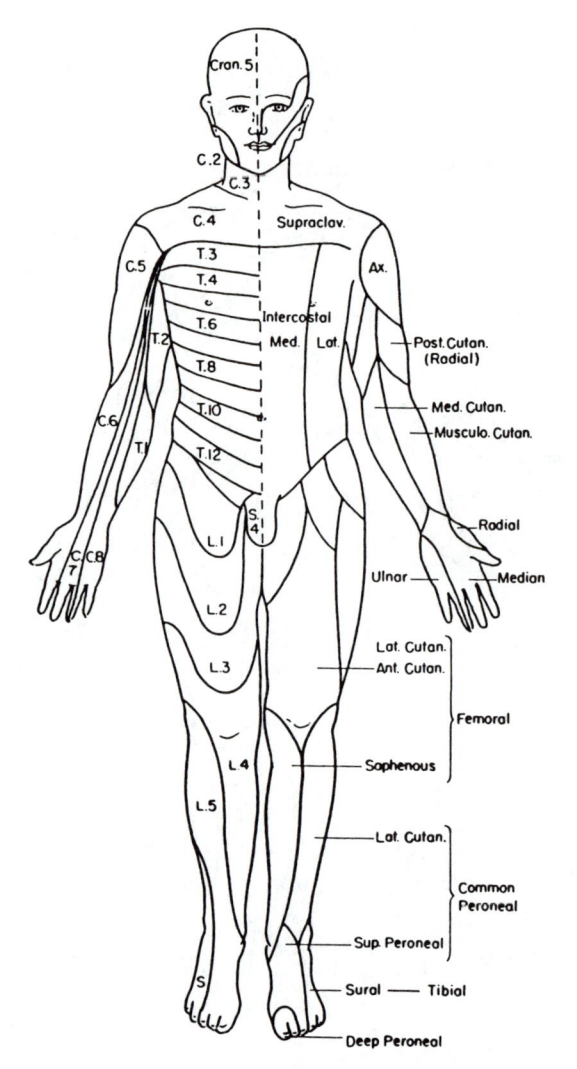

Fig. 3-8

Sensory Dermatomes (Anterior)

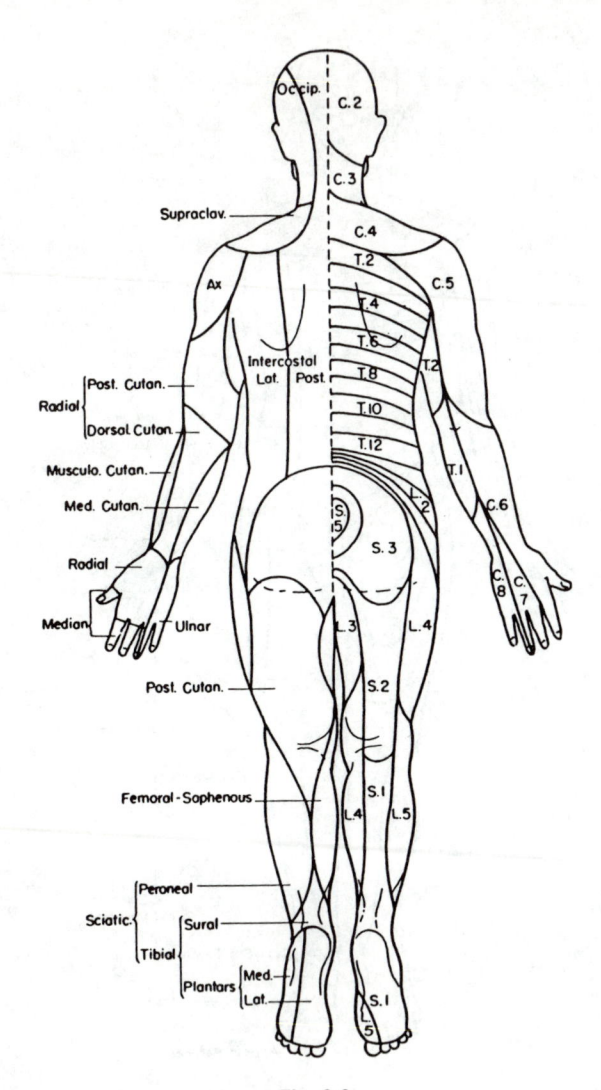

Fig. 3-9

Sensory Dermatomes (Posterior)

hand is rested palm up upon a table to maintain stability. The calipers are placed just lateral to the midline on the finger pad of the distal phalanx. The pressure used on the calipers is enough to just blanch the skin. The patient should then be asked to distinguish between "one" or "two" points. Unaffected or contralateral digits should be examined to gain patient confidence and to determine the normal discrimination for the patient. If the patient is able to discriminate between the two points of the caliper, the distance between the two points should be decreased and the process repeated. The distance is measured for each side of the digit, ulnar and radial. The normal distance for two point discrimination in adults is 6 mm less. See Fig. 3-10.

Specific Examinations and Special Maneuvers

Cervical Spine:[1,9,10]   An examination of the upper extremity should always include an examination of the cervical spine. There are many reports of nerve compression at the foramina and at the carpal tunnel which are unsuccessfully treated with a carpal tunnel release, the so-called <u>double-crush syndrome</u>. In any injury to the upper extremity, a minimum of a cursory exam of the cervical spine is warranted. The patient should be asked to flex his head to the chest, and the distance between the chin and chest should be noted. The patient should then be asked to fully extend his head, and the amount of extension should be noted. Do not confuse extension of the cervical spine with head rotation. At no time should the examiner force the C-spine into position. Rotation and lateral bending of the cervical spine should then be examined by asking the patient to touch his chin and subsequently his ear to his shoulder.

Palpation of the cervical spine should include posterior palpation of the spinous processes as well as anterolateral palpation of the transverse processes. Excessive tenderness should be noted. Palpation of the anterior C-spine should include the lymphatic chain of the supraclavicular region. After the bony landmarks of the C-spine have been palpated, the examiner should examine the surrounding musculature of the neck. Specific attention should be paid to the upper trapezius and the sternocleidomastoid. These muscles are often exquisitely tender after hyperextension (whiplash) injuries. No examination of the cervical spine is complete without documentation of the deep tendon reflexes.

Upper Extremity

Shoulder:[1,9] The shoulder complex consists of the glenohumeral joint, acromioclavicular joint, the sternoclavicular joint, and the articulation of the scapula with the thorax. This joint has the largest range of motion of any joint in the body and is relatively superficial. The glenohumeral articulation is very small to allow for the large range of motion. The stability of the joint is provided by the soft tissues that surround the joint.

Ulnar Nerve
Zone of
Autonomous
Innervation
(Volar)

Median Nerve zone
of Autonomous
Innervation
(Volar)

Radial Nerve Zone of
Autonomous Innervation
(Dorsal)

Fig. 3-10

Zones of Autonomous Innervation for Testing the Nerves Supplying the Hand

The shoulder is easily palpated, and significant landmarks include the acromioclavicular joint, the clavicle, the spine of the scapula, the bicipital groove of the humerus, and the acromion. The examination should begin with a visual inspection to determine abnormal contours or variance with the opposite shoulder. Observation and palpation of the acromioclavicular joint is a critical part of the examination to rule out acromioclavicular injury or arthritis.

Initial examination should include palpation of the bony skeleton and the shoulder girdle musculature. Specific attention should be addressed to the deltoid, the pectorals, the long head of the biceps, and the rotator cuff musculature.

The rotator cuff is susceptible to damage, and several specific tests have been developed to examine this muscle group. The rotator cuff musculature forms a sleeve around the humeral head. These muscles serve as abductors and external rotators of the shoulder. Tears in the rotator cuff usually occur between the insertion of the supraspinatus and the subscapularis. These tears often propagate along the tendons of these muscles medially. By extending the shoulder, a portion of the humeral head can be palpated where the rotator cuff inserts. Pain in this region is suggestive of a rotator cuff tear, but patients with subacromial bursitis will often have pain in this region. The "drop-arm" test examines the rotator cuff. Have the patient abduct his arm to 90 degrees and then ask him to lower his arm to his side slowly while the examiner applies gentle pressure. At approximately 30 degrees of abduction, the patient will no longer be able to gradually lower his arm and it will fall to the side. Unfortunately, the test is not always specific for a rotator cuff tear.

Shoulder impingement is also a common cause of chronic shoulder pain.[13,15] This may or may not be associated with a rotator cuff tear. This is caused by hypertrophy of the acromion and impingement of the humeral head on the acromion. This can be tested by having the patient place his hand on the unaffected shoulder and gradually forward flexing the shoulder. If this motion is painful at 90 degrees of forward flexion it is a positive sign for impingement.

Elbow:[1,9] The elbow is a ginglymus or hinge joint. The normal range of motion of the elbow in the adult is 0-145 degrees in the adult. On initial examination of a patient with elbow pain, the elbow should be examined for its carrying angle. The carrying angle is the amount of valgus with the elbow in full extension. This averages approximately 11 degrees with considerable variation about the mean. Males tend to have smaller carrying angles (5-10 degrees), and females have larger angles (10-15 degrees). The medial collateral ligament is the major stabilizer of the elbow against valgus stress, while the radial head is the secondary stabilizer. Significant deviations from the normal carrying angle is usually the result of a physeal injury or fracture malunion during growth. Examination of the carrying angle with the elbow in less than full extension can lead to false measurements. The carrying angle is rarely a functional problem; however, it can be a cosmetic problem. The elbow has a complex articulation, and the range of motion examination should include flexion-extension and pronation-supination measurements.

There are a number of significant landmarks that are easily palpated in the elbow. Laterally, the landmarks that are easily palpated include the lateral epicondyle and the radial head. Posteriorly, the major landmark is the olecranon, which is the site of insertion of the triceps. Just medial to the olecranon is the ulnar groove in the humerus, which contains the ulnar nerve. Medially, the medial supracondylar line of the humerus can be palpated beneath the wrist flexor insertions. The medial epicondyle of the humerus lies distally on the medial aspect of the elbow. Palpation of the triangle formed between the olecranon posteriorly and the olecranon and epicondyle laterally will often demonstrate an effusion if one is present. These are also the landmarks for comparison with the opposite elbow and for arthrocentesis when it is indicated.

In the child, the most common injury to the elbow is the nursemaid's elbow.[14] The patient is usually a toddler who sustains the injury by having the arm forcefully pulled in extension. The mechanism of the injury is a subluxation of the radial head over the annulus. Since there is not a frank dislocation, there will be no findings on radiographic examination. The child will not be using the extremity, and will have pain on palpation of the radial head. Any attempt at flexion of the elbow will cause pain. The subluxation can be reduced be gentle distraction of the extremity with the arm initially in extension and supination. While the distraction is maintained, the arm is brought into flexion and pronation with downward pressure on the radial head. Often, a click will be heard or felt when the subluxation is reduced. After the reduction, the child will begin to use the extremity again.

In the mature skeleton, the most common fracture is a fracture of the radial head. The history is usually a fall onto the elbow with some initial minimal pain. In nondisplaced fractures, the trauma is usually not great, and the patient will describe a gradual increase in discomfort and a decrease in ROM. These patients usually present some hours after injury with a painful elbow and limited ROM. The elbow will be held in flexion and neutral rotation or slight supination. Palpation of the joint will demonstrate a tense effusion. Radiologic examination of the elbow will demonstrate the presence of an anterior and posterior fat pad sign with or without evidence of fracture. The presence of a posterior fat pad sign is considered diagnostic for a radial head fracture in the presence of no obvious bony injury. Management of the nondisplaced fracture is strictly symptomatic with arthrocentesis of the joint and immobilization for comfort with early range of motion.[15]

Hand and Wrist:[1,2,3,9] Examination of the hand is extremely complex. The examination can only be as thorough as the examiner's knowledge of the anatomy and biomechanics.

The bony architecture of the hand consists of the distal radius and ulna, the eight carpals, five metacarpals, and 14 phalanges. Sensation is supplied by three nerves. The radial nerve supplies the radial-dorsal aspect; the median nerve supplies the thumb, index, and long fingers; and the ulnar nerve supplies sensation to the ring and little fingers (note: there can be considerable overlap of the innervated areas) (Fig. 3-10). Major muscle groups can be divided by both location (intrinsic and extrinsic) and function.

Prominent bony landmarks that can be palpated include the radial styloid, the scaphoid (carpal navicular), trapezium, and first metacarpal along the radial border of the hand. On the radial palmar aspect of the wrist, the tuberosity of the scaphoid can be palpated. On the dorsal aspect of the radius is Lister's tubercle. Distal to Lister's tubercle, the depression of the capitate can be palpated. Along the ulnar side of the wrist and hand, the ulnar styloid and the triquetrum can be palpated. The pisiform bone lies in the tendon of the flexor carpi ulnaris.

Examination of the hand should include measurement of the range of motion of the wrist and digits. Care should be taken to isolate each digit when testing for motor strength or active range of motion. Sensory testing should include the autonomous zones of innervation for each nerve, as well as two-point discrimination (Fig. 3-10).

Specific tests of the hand include testing for thumb adduction by asking the patient to pinch with the thumb tip to the side of the index finger. If the patient has a weak adductor pollicis muscle, which is innervated by the ulnar nerve, the interphalangeal joint of the thumb will flex, as adduction is performed by the flexor musculature of the thumb. The hyperflexion of the thumb IP joint with pinch is known as Froment's sign. An excellent test for ulnar nerve function is to ask the patient to cross his fingers. This ability is limited or absent in a patient with a nonfunctioning ulnar nerve.

The extrinsic finger musculature should also be tested as follows. The extensor digitorum communis (EDC) is tested by asking the patient to extend the MCPJ with the PIPJ flexed to eliminate the action of the intrinsics in extending the distal joints of the digits. The flexor digitorum profundi (FDP) are tested by having the patient flex the DIPJ while the examiner holds the PIPJ fully extended (Fig. 3-11). The flexor digitorum superficialis (FDS) is tested by asking the patient to flex the digit while the examiner holds the contiguous digits fully extended (Fig. 3-12).

The intrinsic musculature of the hand is examined as follows. The opponens pollicis is tested by asking the patient to touch the tip of his thumb to the tip of each digit. The adductor pollicis is tested by asking the patient to tighten his thumb against his index finger in the first web space, or to hold an object tightly between the two fingers in that web space. The lumbricals and interossei are tested by asking the patient to flex the MCPJ while holding the PIPJ and DIPJ fully extended. The interossei are also tested by asking the patient to spread all his fingers against pressure.

Compression of the median nerve at the wrist commonly occurs with flexor tenosynovitis. There are several maneuveurs that can be used to demonstrate compression at the transverse carpal ligament. Percussion of the ligament will cause paresthesias in the median nerve distribution in the affected patient. This is known as Tinel's sign. Phalen's test is performed by flexing the wrists completely for one minute. If the patient develops symptoms of carpal tunnel syndrome before this time expires the test is positive for compression of

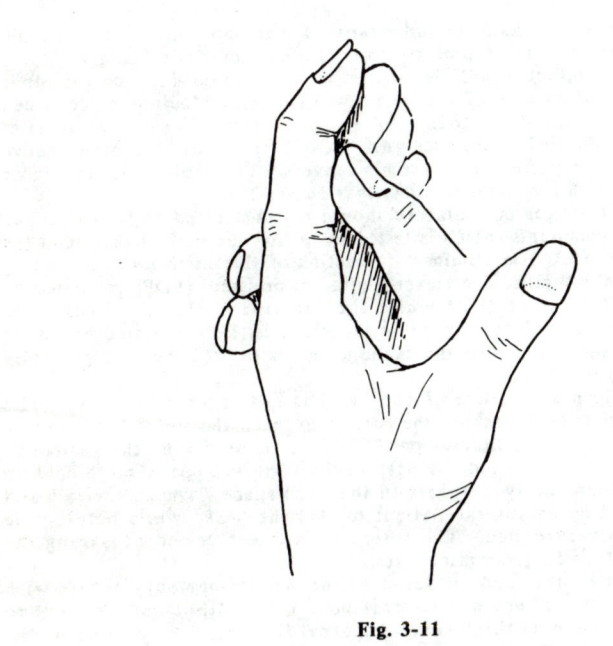

Fig. 3-11

Testing the Index Finger FDP

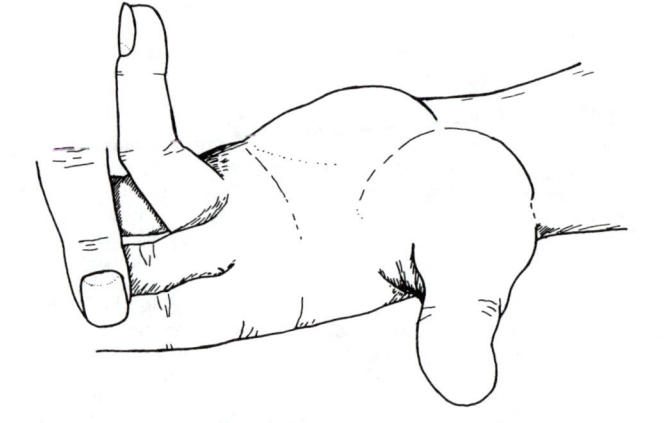

Fig. 3-12

Testing the Ring Finger FDS

the median nerve at the wrist. Carpal tunnel syndrome can produce pain along the entire nerve distribution. There is a well-described entity of the <u>double-crush syndrome</u> where the nerve can be compressed at two separate sites.

Lower Extremity

Pelvis and Hip:[1,9] The pelvis functions as a bony structure to transfer axial forces from the lower extremity to the spine. The pelvis is formed from the coalescence of three bones: the ilium, the ischium, and the pubis. The junction of the these three bones forms the triradiate cartilage in the child, which will eventually fuse and form the acetabulum. The femur is the longest bone in the body and the proximal portion of the femur articulates with the acetabulum in a ball and socket joint.

Anteriorly on the pelvis, significant landmarks include the anterior superior iliac spine, the iliac crest, the pubic tubercles, and the symphysis pubis. Posteriorly, the landmarks include the posterior superior iliac spine, the iliac crest, and the ischial tuberosity. The greater trochanter is the only palpable landmark of the proximal femur. Palpation of these landmarks can be extremely difficult in the obese patient. When palpating the hip and pelvis, the relationship of the greater trochanter to the pelvis should be checked to confirm the location of the femoral head in the acetabulum. Pain over the sacroiliac joints may be the only clinical evidence for sacroiliac (SI) joint ligamentous injury in light of a normal radiograph. In the trauma patient, the pelvis should be checked for stability by attempting to compress the iliac wings and noting any patient discomfort.

The range of motion of the hip is examined in all planes. This should include abduction, adduction, flexion, and extension. Internal and external rotation of the femur should be checked with the hip both flexed to 90 degrees and fully extended. When testing the passive range of motion, the examiner should stabilize the pelvis so true hip motion is tested. In patients with osteoarthritis of the hip, the first limitation in range of motion is in internal rotation.

The gait pattern will often give extensive information about disease of the hip, although gait disturbances can be caused by injury to any joint in the lower extremity, as well as injury to the lumbosacral spine. When examining the gait, observe one portion of the gait at a time. Specific notation should be made of any support the patient uses (i.e., crutch, cane, or walker). With the patient standing, leg length should be examined by palpating the iliac crests posteriorly. Care should be taken to ensure that the knee is fully extended, as a bent knee will contribute to an apparent limb length discrepancy. If a limb length discrepancy is present, the most accurate method of measuring the discrepancy is by placing wooden blocks of standard sizes under the short leg.

Trendelenburg test: This test examines the strength of the gluteus medius. In the normal patient, the pelvis is level when the patient stands. When the patient is asked to stand on one leg, the gluteus medius on the supported side contracts and the pelvis will remain level or elevate on the unsupported side. If the pelvis cannot be maintained level on the unsupported side, the patient is said to have a "positive" Trendelenburg sign. Patients with gluteus medius weakness walk with a limp or lurch on the affected side. This gait pattern is described as Trendelenburg gait. A Trendelenburg gait will be present in almost any painful condition of the hip joint as well as in cases of gluteus medius weakness.

Thomas test: This maneuver is used to determine if a fixed flexion contracture of the hip is present. The examiner locks the pelvis by bringing the contralateral leg into maximal flexion with the patient supine on the examining table. This causes the pelvis to rotate forward and eliminate the lumbar lordosis. (Excessive lumbar lordosis can be used to compensate for a hip flexion contracture.) The leg to be examined is then brought into maximal extension with the hip in slight adduction and internal rotation. If the leg does not fully extend to touch the examining table, then a fixed flexion contracture is present, and the angle of the flexion contracture can be estimated by measuring the lack of extension of the limb to touch the table.

Ober's test:[11,16] Since the widespread use of the polio vaccine, the incidence of iliotibial band contracture has decreased. The Ober test measures the amount of abduction contracture caused by the iliotibial band. The patient is placed on his side with the affected limb on the top. The pelvis is again locked by bringing the unaffected limb into maximal flexion. The affected limb is then brought into full extension and abduction. From the position of abduction, the leg is allowed to fall into adduction. If a contracture is present, the affected limb will not be able to move into adduction. In performing the test, the leg must be brought into full extension to place the iliotibial band over the greater trochanter. If the iliotibial band is permitted to move anterior to the greater trochanter, the test will yield a false-negative result.

Knee: The knee is one of the most commonly injured joints. Much of the diagnosis of soft tissue pathology in the knee is made on the basis of the clinical examination. If the patient presents rapidly for assessment after an acute injury, tests for instability can be performed with minimal patient discomfort. In the presence of a tense knee effusion, performing an anterior drawer test can border on torture for the unanesthesized patient.

The knee consists of the articulations between the tibia and the distal femur. The femur has two articulations, which are the medial and lateral condyles. The tibia has a proximal flare or plateau which is divided into medial and lateral compartments by the intercondylar tubercle. The articulations between the tibia and femur contain both articular and meniscal cartilage.

Landmarks of the knee include the tibial tubercle and the patella anteriorly. The adductor tubercle is palpable on the medial femoral condyle. Posteriorly, the neurovascular bundle is found in the popliteal fossa between the insertions of the gastrocnemius. Gerdy's tubercle is palpable on the lateral tibia. Other anatomic structures include the insertion of the pes anserinus (sartorius, gracilis, and semitendinosus tendons) on the medial tibia, the insertion of the medial and lateral hamstrings on the tibia and fibula respectively, and the iliotibial band which is palpated laterally before its insertion at Gerdy's tubercle. The quadriceps tendon can be palpated superior to the patella, and it extends to its insertion on the tibial tubercle as the patellar tendon. The medial and lateral collateral ligaments are located on the respective sides of the knee. Pain over the origins of these ligaments with valgus and varus stress respectively can be associated with strain or rupture of these structures.

The presence or absence of an effusion is helpful in the diagnosis of a knee injury. There are also several bursae surrounding the knee which may give rise to localized swelling. In addition, the effusion may be chronic or acute. The easiest way to demonstrate an effusion is to "milk" the effusion from the suprapatellar pouch into the infrapatellar region where it will be appreciated as a fullness medial and lateral to the patellar tendon. The joint is milked by pressing on the suprapatellar area, and sliding the hand distally. In a large effusion, the patella may be ballotable against the femoral condyles. This is performed by depressing the patella into the trochlear groove and then releasing it - the displaced effusion will cause the patella to rebound.

The majority of injuries to the knee are to soft tissue, although radiographs of the knee should be made to examine the bony architecture. For instance, in some anterior cruciate tears, the ligament is avulsed from the bony origin or insertion with a small fragment of bone. The avulsion of the ligamentous insertion has prognostic significance in that a primary repair can be performed.

The major ligaments involved in knee injuries include the medial and lateral collateral ligaments which are extraarticular, and the anterior and posterior cruciate ligaments, which are intraarticular. Many injuries to the major ligaments of the knee will be associated with injury to the meniscal cartilage, as these are secondary stabilizers of the knee.

An examination of the knee should begin by palpation of the knee joint. The localization of pain is often diagnostic. The active and passive range of motion of the joint should be documented. Tenderness along the joint line either medially or laterally should suggest a meniscal injury. Pain over Gerdy's tubercle is often associated with inflammation of the iliotibial band, known as <u>iliotibial band syndrome</u>. Lateral knee pain with the affected leg placed in the figure-four position is often associated with lateral collateral ligament injury. If range of motion is limited, its etiology should be determined. A locked knee can be caused by a meniscal tear or a cruciate ligament subluxed into the joint. Lack of full extension can be caused by an anterior meniscal lesion. Pain with flexion of the knee can be associated with posterior horn meniscal tears (these are commonly seen in football lineman and powerlifting). Limitation of active extension can be caused by injury to the extensor mechanism, specifically a patella fracture, patellar tendon rupture, or quadriceps tendon rupture.

Drawer tests:[7,17] The drawer test examines the knee for instability of the cruciate ligaments. The anterior drawer tests the anterior cruciate, and the posterior drawer evaluates the posterior cruciate. To perform the anterior drawer test, have the patient lie in the supine position with the knee flexed 90 degrees and the foot flat on the examining table in the neutral position. Encircle the tibia with both hands, and place the thumbs on the anterior surface just below the joint line. The foot is stabilized on the table by bracing it with the examiner's hip. With the patient relaxed, attempt to pull the tibia forward on the femur. If the tibia moves forward without a definite stopping point, the anterior cruciate may be damaged. In the normal population, there may be some laxity, so comparison of findings should be made with the uninjured knee. This test is not valid if the quadriceps and hamstrings are not relaxed. In the acutely injured patient, it may not be possible to perform this test secondary to patient discomfort. The posterior drawer test is performed in the same fashion, although pressure is applied to the anterior portion of the tibia in an attempt to sublux the tibia posteriorly.

External and internal rotation of the foot in conjunction with the anterior drawer test can give information about the posteromedial and posterolateral capsular stability, respectively. The posteromedial knee capsule tightens with the foot in external rotation, and the anterior drawer should be less even in the presence of a torn anterior cruciate. If the amount of forward motion is the same as with the foot in neutral postion, posteromedial capsule damage can be suspected. With the foot in internal rotation, the posterolateral structures tighten, and the amount of forward motion with the anterior drawer test should be diminished despite an anterior cruciate injury. Again, if forward motion is the same as when the foot is in the neutral position, there may be injury to the posterolateral capsule.

Lachman's test:[7,17] Lachman's test is another test for stability of the anterior cruciate ligament. This test can be performed with a minimum of discomfort on the acutely injured knee in the presence of an effusion. The test is performed with the patient in the supine postion. The examiner supports the leg under his arm with his contralateral arm beneath the tibia. The examiner's other hand is placed just medial to the patellar tendon with one digit palpating the tibia, and another palpating the medial femoral condyle. With the patient as relaxed as possible, the examiner attempts to bring the tibia forward on the femur. Any motion of the joint will be seen and felt by the examiner. Again, the key to a successful assessment is relaxation of the musculature. Any findings should be compared with the contralateral limb.

Varus and valgus stress:[7] The medial collateral ligament (MCL) can be tested by applying forced valgus stress on the limb. With the patient supine, the leg to be examined is supported under the proximal tibia by the examiner's contralateral hand. With the knee flexed 10-15 degrees, a valgus force is applied gradually to the knee joint with the other hand. If the MCL is injured, the patient will have pain in the anatomic region which will increase with stress. Using the same method, a varus force is applied to the knee to test the lateral collateral ligament.

Pivot shift:[7,17] The femoral condyle is shaped in the form of a cam. Motion at the knee joint is a combination of rotation and gliding of the femoral condyle over the tibia. In the presence of an anterior cruciate deficiency, there is excessive anterior gliding of the tibia. The pivot shift test examines the motion of the knee as it goes from flexion to full extension. If excessive gliding is present, there will be excessive anterior motion of the lateral femoral condyle on the lateral tibial plateau as it "screws home" near terminal extension. This test is performed with the patient supine, and the knee held in flexion by the examiner, who also places a valgus/internal rotation stress to the knee. The knee is extended by the examiner, and the lateral joint line palpated. If the lateral femoral joint line demonstrates excessive anterior motion, then the test is stated to be positive. This test is difficult to perform, and findings with the test should be correlated with other portion of the exam.

McMurray test:[9] This test examines the knee for a tear in the posterior horn of the medial meniscus. The test is performed with the patient supine, and the knee flexed. The foot is internally and externally rotated to loosen the knee joint. The knee is then brought into extension with the foot held in external rotation and a steady valgus force applied. If a click or pop is appreciated during extension, the test is suggestive for a posterior medial meniscus tear.

Foot and Ankle:[1,9] The foot and ankle are a complex series of bones, joints, and soft tissues which require a great deal of skill and experience to examine. Examination begins by inspecting and comparing the two feet to determine any asymmetry between them.

After inspecting the feet, the foot and ankle are palpated to determine any areas of tenderness. The palpation should proceed along well-known anatomic landmarks and should include the lateral and medial malleolus, the talar head, the deltoid ligament, the anterior talofibular ligament, and the sustentaculum tali (along the medial aspect of the calcaneus).

Range of motion of the foot and ankle should next be determined. As the foot consists of multiple joints, it is almost impossible to examine each joint for range of motion, while separating the motions from that of contiguous joints and recording it accurately. More commonly, range of motion is recorded of the following aspects of the foot and ankle: dorsi- and plantarflexion of the talocrural (ankle) joint, inversion and eversion of the subtalar joint (performed by stabilizing the talus in the ankle mortise with one hand while testing motion of the subtalar joint with the other hand), motion of the midfoot (the talonavicular and calcaneocuboid joints - tested by stabilizing the heel with one hand and testing eversion and inversion, and adduction and abduction of the forefoot with the other hand), and motion of the first ray, noting dorsi- and plantarflexion at the metatarsophalangeal and interphalangeal joint.

Motion can be recorded both passively and actively. More commonly, it is measured passively by the examiner. However, active motion is also tested during the muscle testing portion of the foot and ankle exam. The following muscles are usually tested: ankle plantarflexion (gastrocsoleus complex), ankle dorsiflexion (peroneals and anterior tibial), foot eversion (peroneals), foot inversion (anterior and posterior tibial), toe extension (extensor digitorum longus and extensor hallucis longus), and toe flexion (flexor digitorum longus and brevis). In addition to providing information about each individual muscle, this portion of the exam may help identify any problems relating to lumbar nerve roots as the muscle groups are innervated by specific nerve roots (Tables 3-2 and 3-3).

In cases of acute or chronic ankle sprains specific tests of the foot and ankle include the anterior and posterior drawer tests and inversion stress tests. These test, respectively, the anterior talofibular ligament (ATFL), the posterior talofibular ligament (PTFL), and the calcaneofibular ligament (CFL). These are the three ligaments usually involved in inversion ankle sprains, with the ATFL the most commonly injured. The CFL is injured or torn in severe ankle sprains, while the PTFL is rarely torn.

The anterior drawer test is the most important of the three tests. It is performed by stabilizing the distal tibia with one hand, while the opposite hand grasps the hindfoot. The hand about the hindfoot should hold it laterally, with two or three fingers around the back of the calcaneus and the thumb over the dorsolateral aspect of the foot. As the distal tibia is stabilized, an attempt is made to bring the hindfoot forward on the tibia, while also slightly internally rotating it. Any significant forward slide relative to the opposite, normal ankle, is termed a positive anterior drawer sign and is indicative of damage to the ATFL. The posterior drawer is performed with the hands in the same position, except that the motion is an attempt to posteriorly displace the hindfoot relative to the tibia.

The inversion stress test is performed by stabilizing the tibia with one hand while the palm of the other hand cups the plantar aspect of the hindfoot.

As the tibia is stabilized, the opposite hand attempts to invert the hindfoot underneath the ankle mortise. The result is compared to the opposite, normal foot to assess any damage to the calcaneo-fibular ligament.

The Pediatric Examination[4,5,11,16]

Examination of children is not simply the examination of a smaller-sized version of an adult. Children are different both physiologically and psychologically, and the differences must be borne in mind. Although it is always a good idea to examine the "normal" extremity when one is presented with a unilateral complaint, this notion is of paramount importance in children in order to establish some trust between the child and the examiner. Failure to do so, and immediate examination of the injured, painful area, will result only in pain and distrust for the child, and frustration for the examiner and the parents. After examining the normal extremity, the examination of the injured limb should begin in an area which is not injured and only at the end of the exam should the injured area be palpated and examined.

Neonates have certain musculoskeletal differences which change gradually as the child grows. Many of the initial differences are related to positioning of the fetus in the uterus. In order to understand what is normal and abnormal in children, it is absolutely necessary to understand the varying growth patterns of the extremities in children.

It is also important to obtain a good history about developmental landmarks. This helps assess neurologic development. The parents should be questioned about when the child first began to sit up, to crawl, to attempt to stand, and to walk. Normal milestones are approximately as follows:[5,11,16]

Head control - about 3 months
Sitting independently - about 6 months
Crawling - about 8 months
Pulling to stand - about 10 months
Walking independently - about 12 months

The neonatal spine has a long, kyphotic C-curve with no areas of lordosis initially present. This is because of the "curled up" position which the child assumed in the womb. As children grow and begin to sit and raise their heads, the spine will develop the normal lumbar and cervical lordosis. The cervical lordosis develops as the child begins to raise his head, at about 2-3 months, while the lumbar curve is well developed when the child is sitting up and beginning to stand, usually by 10-12 months.

The neonatal spine must also be examined to be certain there are no skin defects, skin discoloration, or hair tufts. All of these are suggestive of spinal dysraphism, such as myelomeningocoele or diastamatomyelia.

In utero the fetal upper extremity is usually positioned with the arms across the chest and the elbows flexed. Thus, most neonates have flexion contractures at the elbows and slight internal rotation contractures of the shoulders. These correct as the child begins to use his hands and should be fully corrected by 6 months to one year of age.

In the newborn, the most important musculoskeletal assessment is the hip joint. The developing femoral head must be directed toward the developing acetabulum (triradiate cartilage). The incidence of instability of the hip in the newborn has been reported as one in 60 by Barlow. Early detection of hip instability will often allow for simple closed management of the problem with minimal late sequelae.

The child should be examined when he/she is cooperative. Little information will be gained from the examination of a crying six-month-old. All examinations of the hip should be made with the child entirely disrobed, including removal of the diaper. With the child in the supine position and the legs extended, the skin should be examined for asymmetric skin folds as well as any other gross abnormality.

With the pelvis level on the examining table, the knees should be brought together with the hips flexed 90 degrees. A dislocation should be suspected if there is an apparent discrepancy in leg length with the affected side being shorter (pediatric hip dislocations are typically lateral and superior). This assessment of leg length is known as Galeazzi's sign.

Ortolani's test:[4,11,16] With the child in the supine position and the hips flexed 90 degrees, the distal femur is controlled by the thumb, and the fingers are placed over the greater trochanter. The hip is then slowly abducted. If the hip is dislocated, the examiner will feel a click as the hip relocates into the acetabulum. A helpful mnemonic for recalling the postion of the femoral head is that in Ortolani's test the femoral head starts "out" and is reduced "in." OUT-IN, O-I, O-rtolan-I.

Barlow's test:[4,11,16] This test is essentially the opposite of the Ortolani test, as here an unstable hip is dislocated out of the acetabulum. The test is performed by bringing the hip into adduction with gentle axial pressure. An instability will be felt as a click as the femoral head subluxes over the rim of the acetabulum.

Nelaton's line:[11,16] The presence of the greater trochanter above a line between the anterior superior iliac spine and the ischial tuberosity signifies a dislocation of the hip.

The child should then be placed in the prone position, and the amount of internal and external rotation of the hip should be measured. These ranges of motion should be symmetric. A discrepancy between each leg should make the examiner suspicious for dislocation. With the child supine, abduction of each hip with the hips flexed 90 degrees should also be compared. Again, asymmetry between the hips is very suggestive of a hip dislocation.

All normal neonates are born with hip flexion contractures of about 30 degrees. The absence of a hip flexion contracture is an excellent indication of a congenital dislocation of the hip. Hip extension must be tested with the opposite hip flexed fully to stabilize the pelvis.

With the child supine, the hips should be internally and externally rotated, with the hips both extended and flexed. In adults, the hips internally rotate less than they externally rotate. Neonates usually have a slight external rotation contracture. However, this is compensated by the fact that the femoral neck is anteverted more in children than it is in adults. (Anteversion measures the relationship of the femoral neck to the knee axis.) As the child begins to stand, the external rotation contracture stretches out and the excessive anteversion causes the child to stand with the legs slightly internally rotated and the toes thus pointing in a bit - "toeing-in."

Toeing-in is a common reason for parents to bring their child to clinic, and femoral anteversion is the most common cause of toeing-in. However, as the child learns to walk, the femoral anteversion usually corrects to normal adult values (about 15 degrees) and the child will eventually walk with the toes pointing relatively straight ahead. Rarely is surgery required for excessive femoral anteversion. Bracing has not been shown to improve this condition, so the parents should usually be reassured that this is normal physiologic development and corrects in most instances.

The knee examination in children is usually performed when anxious parents bring the child to clinic concerned about knock-knees (genu valgum) or bowlegs (genu varum). Virtually all children will have genu varum when they first begin to stand. This usually corrects at about age 2-3, and most children then develop genu valgum until they are about 4-5. Again, this usually corrects to a normal physiologic appearance.

Two causes of severe bowing at the knees are rickets and Blount's disease.[11,16] To eliminate rickets as an etiology, a good nutritional history should be obtained from the parents about how the child is fed. If rickets is suspected, appropriate blood and urine tests can be performed to diagnose it. Blount's disease is a growth disorder of the proximal tibial physis which results in severe genu varum. It usually also presents with a varus thrust during gait and requires radiographic confirmation for accurate diagnosis. Except in moderate-to-severe cases of rickets or Blount's disease, genu varum and valgum rarely require bracing or surgery.

A second common cause of toeing-in is internal tibial torsion. Tibial torsion measures the relationship of the knee axis to the ankle axis and can be determined by flexing the knee, aligning the patella to be directed anteriorly, and then comparing the angle between the lateral and medial malleolus to that of the thigh. Normally, the ankle is externally rotated about 25 degrees relative to the knee and the femur. Less than this would indicate some degree of internal tibial torsion and the foot would point in or toe-in. The opposite problem, toeing-out and external tibial torsion, occurs less frequently.

Because of fetal positioning, many children demonstrate minor degrees of internal tibial torsion when they first begin to stand. This usually corrects after they have been walking for awhile. As with femoral anteversion, surgery is rarely required for this condition, and bracing has not been shown to be of benefit. The parents should be reassured that this is a normal physiologic variant which usually corrects.

Children's feet can have many abnormalities. The most common severe abnormality is a clubfoot, or talipes equinovarus. This is manifested by the foot being plantarflexed (equinus) and turned inward (varus). This condition, if untreated, can cause severe difficulties with walking, as well as pain and degenerative arthritis as the child grows. Mild cases of clubfeet can be treated by serial cast correction, but severe cases require surgical release. However, even severe cases are usually treated by a few months of serial casting to stretch out the soft tissues in preparation for surgical correction.

Another common problem in children's feet is metatarsus adductus. This occurs when the forefoot turns slightly inward, and is another cause of toeing-in. This can be evaluated by examining the plantar aspect of the foot. A midfoot line drawn between the hindfoot and midfoot, if extended anteriorly, should pass between the second and third toes. If this line passes lateral to that web space, metatarsus adductus is present. Another indication of severe metatarsus adductus is the presence of a plantar-medial skin crease. Mild metatarsus adductus can be treated simply by having the parents stretching the feet several times a day. Moderate metatarsus adductus is often treated with reverse-last shoes, i.e., wearing shoes on the opposite feet. Severe metatarsus adductus is usually treated with serial cast correction.

One of the most important aspects of the children's exam consists in simply asking them to walk, as a great deal can be learned from observing the gait. One should observe the child's balance, and note any unusual aspects of the gait, as well as observe the function of the various muscle groups about the foot to determine if any muscles are out of phase during either the swing or stance phase.

Finally, the pediatric examination should include a detailed neurologic evaluation. While it is important to test the strength of the various muscle groups, this is not always possible to do in children because they cannot follow instructions well. In these cases, information can be gained by watching the child play or hold objects, to see which muscle groups appear to be active. In addition, the foot can be stimulated by stroking the plantar surface and seeing which muscles react to pull the foot away from this noxious stimulus.

The neurologic examination includes testing of the deep tendon reflexes, as in the adult. Babinski testing and testing for clonus should be performed. The presence of hyperreflexia, clonus, a stretch reflex (often termed claspknife rigidity) and/or upgoing toes on the Babinski test are the four hallmarks of spasticity and will support a diagnosis of spastic cerebral palsy.

In addition, in the child there are certain infantile reflexes that should be tested if there is any suspicion of a developmental delay. If any two of these reflexes are abnormal after 12 months of age, the prognosis for unassisted ambulation is poor.[5] The infantile reflexes are as follows: Moro reflex, head-turning reflex, asymmetric tonic neck reflex, symmetric tonic neck reflex, foot-placement reaction, extensor thrust, and the parachute reaction.[5,11,16]

The Moro reflex is tested by jarring the table, or dropping the infant's head into extension. The Moro reflex is sudden extension or spreading of the upper extremities. This reflex appears by 6 months but should disappear by 12 to 16 months.

The head-turning reflex is tested with the child in the side-lying position. The head is tilted downward and rotated toward the floor. A positive head-turning reflex is present if the lower extremity on the same side flexes at the hip and knee. The asymmetric tonic neck reflex is tested in the supine position. The head is rotated towards one side and the reflex is present if the extremities extend on the face-turned side and flex on the occiput side. The symmetric tonic neck reflex is tested with the child prone. The reflex is present if extension of the head causes extension of the forelimbs and flexion of the hindlimbs. The three neck reflexes should all disappear in the normal infant at about 6 months.

The foot-placement reaction is tested by holding the child with the feet dangling such that they just touch the edge of the examining table. Normal infants will lift the feet and place them on the table. An abnormal reaction is to simply allow the feet to continue to hang loosely.

Extensor thrust is present if, when the child is held in a weightbearing position, the legs extend at the ankle, knees, and hips and adduct and cross.

The parachute reaction is tested by holding the child under their arms and tilting them downward and forward. Normally, the child will extend the upper extremities as if to break the fall. The parachute reaction normally appears at about 9 months of age. It is abnormal if it is not present after that age.

TABLE 3-1 - MUSCLE GRADING[9,10]

GRADE DESCRIPTION

5	Normal
4	Muscle contraction with full range of motion against gravity with some resistance
3	Muscle contraction with full range of motion against gravity
2	Muscle contraction with full range of motion with gravity eliminated
1	Flicker of muscle contraction
0	No activity

TABLE 3-2[8,9,10]

MUSCLE INNERVATION - UPPER EXTREMITY

MUSCLE	PERIPHERAL NERVE	NERVE ROOT
Trapezius	Cranial Nerve 11	Also C_{2-4}?
Rhomboids	Dorsal scapular	C_5
Levator scapulae	Nn. to levator scapulae	C_{3-4}
Pectoralis major	Medial and lateral pectoral	C_5-T_1
Deltoid	Axillary	C_{5-6}
Latissimus dorsi	Thoracodorsal	C_{6-8}
Supraspinatus	Suprascapular	C_{5-6}
Infraspinatus	Suprascapular	C_{5-6}
Teres major	Lower subscapular	C_{5-6}
Teres minor	Axillary	C_{5-6}
Subscapularis	Upper/lower subscapular	C_{5-6}
Brachialis	Musculocutaneous	C_{5-6}
Biceps	Musculocutaneous	C_{5-6}
Triceps	Radial	C_{6-8}
Anconeus	Radial	C_{7-8}
Brachioradialis	Radial	C_{5-6}
ECRL, ECRB	Radial	C_{6-7}
Supinator	Radial [posterior interosseus]	C_{5-6}
AbPL	Radial [posterior interosseus]	C_{6-7}
ECU	Radial [posterior interosseus]	C_{6-8}
EDC	Radial [posterior interosseus]	C_{6-8}
EDQ	Radial [posterior interosseus]	C_{6-8}
EI	Radial [posterior interosseus]	C_{7-8}
EPB	Radial [posterior interosseus]	C_{6-7}
EPL	Radial [posterior interosseus]	C_{7-8}
FCR	Median	C_{6-7}
FCU	Ulnar	C_8-T_1
FDP [index, long]	Median [anterior interosseus]	C_7-T_1
FDP [ring, little]	Ulnar	C_7-T_1
FDS	Median	C_7-T_1
FPL	Median [anterior interosseus]	C_7-T_1
Pronator teres	Median	C_{6-7}
Pronator quadratus	Median [anterior interosseus]	C_7-T_1
Dorsal interossei	Ulnar	C_8-T_1
Palmar interossei	Ulnar	C_8-T_1
Lumbricals [index,long]	Median	C_7-T_1
Lumbricals [ring, little]	Ulnar	C_7-T_1
APB	Median	C_8-T_1
FPB	Median/ulnar	C_8-T_1
OpP	Median	C_8-T_1
AdP	Ulnar	C_8-T_1
Hypothenars	Ulnar	C_8-T_1

TABLE 3-3[8,9,10]

MUSCLE INNERVATION - LOWER EXTREMITY

MUSCLE	PERIPHERAL NERVE	NERVE ROOT
Gluteus maximus	Inferior gluteal	L_4-S_1
Gluteus medius	Superior gluteal	L_4-S_1
Gluteus minimus	Superior gluteal	L_4-S_1
Hip external rotators	Nerves to . . .	L_4-S_2
Hip adductors	Obturator/tibial	L_{3-4}
Iliopsoas	Femoral	L_{2-3}
Quadriceps	Femoral	L_{2-4}
Sartorius	Femoral	L_{2-3}
Pectineus	Femoral	L_{2-3}
Semitendinosus	Sciatic [tibial]	L_5-S_1
Semimembranosus	Sciatic [tibial]	L_5-S_1
Biceps femoris	Sciatic [tibial/peroneal]	L_5-S_1
Tibialis anterior	Deep peroneal	L_{4-5}
Tibialis posterior	Tibial	L_5-S_1
EDL	Deep peroneal	L_{4-5}
EHL	Deep peroneal	L_5
Peroneus longus, brevis	Superficial peroneal	L_5-S_1
Gastrocnemius	Tibial	S_{1-2}
Soleus	Tibial	S_{1-2}
FDL	Tibial	L_5-S_1
FHL	Tibial	L_5-S_1
Foot intrinsics	Medial/lateral plantar [tibial]	L_5-S_2

TABLE 3-4[8,9,10]

DEEP TENDON REFLEXES

MUSCLE	PERIPHERAL NERVE	NERVE ROOT
Biceps	Musculocutaneous	C_5
Brachioradialis	Radial	C_6
Triceps	Radial	C_7
Quadriceps (knee)	Femoral	L_4
Posterior tibialis	Deep peroneal (rarely elicited)	L_5
Gastroc/soleus	Tibial	S_1

TABLE 3-5[8,9,10]

SUPERFICIAL REFLEXES

REFLEX	PERIPHERAL NERVE	NERVE ROOT
Bulbocavernosus	Pudendal	S_{2-4}
Cremasteric	Genitofemoral	L_1
Babinski	Sciatic	S_1

References

1. American Academy of Orthopaedic Surgeons. *Manual of Orthopaedic Surgery*. Chicago: author, 1979.
2. American Society for Surgery of the Hand. *The Hand: Examination and Diagnosis*. Edinburgh: Churchill-Livingstone, 1983.
3. American Society for Surgery of the Hand. *Syllabus - Regional Review Course in Hand Surgery*. Chicago: author, 1985.
4. Barlow TG. Early diagnosis and treatment of congenital dislocation of the hip. **JBJS**, 44B: 292, 1962.
5. Bleck EE. Locomotor prognosis in cerebral palsy. **Develop. Med. Child. Neurol.**, 17: 18, 1975.
6. Crenshaw AH, ed. *Campbell's Operative Orthopaedics*. 7th edition. St. Louis: C. V. Mosby, 1987; p. 2331.
7. Feagin JA Jr, ed. *The Crucial Ligaments*. New York: Churchill-Livingstone, 1988.
8. Hollinshead WH. *Anatomy for Surgeons: Volume 3. The Back and Limbs*. 2nd edition. New York: Harper & Row, 1969.
9. Hoppenfeld S. *Physical Examination of the Spine and Extremities*. New York: Appleton-Century-Crofts, 1976.
10. Hoppenfeld, S. *Orthopaedic Neurology*. New York: Appleton-Century-Crofts, 1979.
11. Lovell WW, Winter RB. *Pediatric Orthopaedics*. Philadelphia: J. B. Lippincott, 1986.
12. Moberg E. "Methods of Examining Sensibility of the Hand," In: Flynn JE, ed. *Hand Surgery*. Baltimore: Williams & Wilkins, 1966.
13. Neer CS II. Impingement lesions. **CORR** 173: 70, 1983.
14. Rockwood CA Jr, Wilkins KE, King RE. *Fractures in Children (Volume 3)*. Philadelphia: J. B. Lippincott, 1984.
15. Rockwood CA Jr, Green DP. *Fractures in Adults (Volume 1)*. Philadelphia: J. B. Lippincott, 1984.
16. Tachdjian MO, ed. *Pediatric Orthopaedics*. Philadelphia: Saunders, 1972.
17. Torg JS, Conrad W, Kalen J. Clinical diagnosis of anterior cruciate ligament instability in the athlete. **Am. J. Sports Med.**, 4: 84, 1976.

Chapter 4

Radiologic Evaluation of the Orthopaedic Patient

Radiographic imaging is a useful, and in many cases necessary, tool in the diagnosis of orthopaedic injuries. Adequate imaging will assist in the diagnosis and subsequent evaluation of reduction maneuvers. The examiner should select the appropriate views so that a diagnosis is not missed.

Special mention is warranted in the examination of the unresponsive trauma patient. Additional screening films are necessary so that occult injuries are not overlooked. These views should always include a minimum of a lateral cervical spine film which includes the cervicothoracic junction, and an anteroposterior view of the pelvis.

Plain Radiographs

Radiographs evaluate the bones in a single plane. In order to adequately evaluate the bony skeleton, the part to be examined should be viewed in a minimum of two planes which are 90 degrees apart. The following paragraphs list the routine views for the evaluation of orthopaedic trauma. These lists are merely introductory guidelines, and additional views including "cone-down," and obliques can yield additional information about fractures.

C-spine: A-P, lateral, open-mouth odontoid, bilateral obliques. The study is not considered adequate unless the cervicothoracic junction is visualized, including the superior portion of the body of T_1.

Trauma C-spine: A-P, lateral, bilateral trauma obliques, odontoid view. These views are obtained with the patient immobilized in the supine position. After interpretation of these films, formal obliques and lateral views are performed with the patient in the upright postion (if the patient can cooperate). If there is any question regarding C-spine injury, immobilization is not removed, and additional imaging is performed using computed or plane tomography. If ligamentous instability is noted in the awake and alert patient, the evaluation progresses with lateral flexion-extension views of the cervical spine. **THE PATIENT MUST FLEX AND EXTEND HIS OWN NECK WITHOUT ASSISTANCE FROM THE PHYSICIAN OR TECHNICIAN.**

Shoulder: For an elective shoulder series, the standard is an A-P view with the arm in internal rotation, an A-P view with the arm in external rotation, and an axillary lateral view. The trauma series includes a true A-P (shot perpendicular to the scapular blade rather than the coronal plane of the body and also termed a glenoid fossa view), a Y-lateral view, and an axillary lateral view. To determine the presence or absence of a Hill-Sachs lesion in the evaluation of shoulder instability, two views often ordered are a Stryker notch and a West Point view.

Clavicle: A-P of shoulder. Fractures of the distal clavicle can be seen on routine views of the shoulder. If additional views are indicated, the tube can be aimed cephalad 40 degrees to isolate the clavicle above the rib cage.

Acromioclavicular Joint: When instability of the acromioclavicular (A-C) joint is suspected, stress views of the A-C joint should be made. These views are an A-P view of the shoulders with both shoulders included on the same film. The view is then repeated with 10 lbs. of weight secured to the patient's wrists. The patient should not hold the weights, as this tenses the shoulder musculature. When imaging this joint, the roentgen beam needs to be angled such that it aims 15 degrees cephalad.

Humerus: A-P, lateral views.

Elbow: A-P and lateral view of the elbow is usually sufficient; however, an oblique view may give additional information about the radial head. When the elbow cannot be fully extended, the A-P view should center on the elbow joint, not the humeral shaft. Elbow films should also include a sufficient amount of the humerus and forearm, so that assessment of alignment can be made.

Wrist: A-P, lateral, and oblique view of the wrist are adequate in most cases. When a distal radius fracture is suspected, the film must contain a sufficient length of the radius to assess the alignment of the fracture in both the lateral and A-P planes. When carpal pathology is seen on routine views or suspected based on clinical examination, six additional views can be helpful. These views include A-P views in maximal radial and ulnar deviation, lateral views in maximal volar and dorsal flexion, and a clenched-fist P-A and lateral.

Hand and Digits: An A-P, lateral and oblique view constitutes the initial examination. When there is damage to a separate digit, a lateral of the specific digit is necessary for the measurement of alignment.

Thoracic Spine: A-P and lateral views.

Lumbosacral Spine: The full series includes seven views: A-P, lateral, bilateral 30 degrees obliques, a coccyx view, a cone-down view of the lumbosacral junction, and an A-P pelvis. When possible, the films should be obtained in the standing position.

Trauma Lumbosacral Series: This includes the above series with specific attention to the thoracolumbar junction. When instability is suspected, lateral flexion and extension views should be obtained.

Scoliosis Series: These films include a P-A and lateral of the spine with left and right lateral bending views shot in a P-A direction. These views should include all curves on a single film (i.e., thoracolumbosacral). Whenever possible, these films should be obtained with the patient in the weightbearing position. P-A projections of lateral bending will yield important preoperative information about curve flexibility. P-A views, as opposed to A-P views, decrease the amount of radiation to the radiosensitive breast and thyroid tissue in the adolescent.

Pelvis: In pelvic trauma, a complete pelvic series includes an A-P view, Judet views (oblique projections with the pelvis rotated 45 degrees), and inlet/outlet views (A-P projections with the tube directed 25 degrees caudad, and 35 degrees cephalad). In acetabular fractures, a computed tomogram (CT) of the pelvis is necessary for an assessment of joint congruity.

Hip: A-P pelvis, A-P hip, and cross table lateral. The lateral view demonstrates the femoral head, and the acetabular articulation. A standing true lateral view of the hip demonstrates the relationship of the femur to the pelvis (pelvic flexion). This view is helpful in the preoperative planning of hip arthroplasty. Another view often performed in a standard series is a frog-leg lateral. This is very useful in pediatric conditions, especially evaluation of Legg-Calvé-Perthes disease and slipped capital femoral epiphyses. However, in the adult or in the trauma patient, it yields minimal information as it provides a lateral of the proximal femur rather than of the pelvis and acetabulum. One exception is that a frog-leg lateral radiograph may be used to evaluate avascular necrosis of the femoral head in the adult.

Knee: A-P, lateral, intercondylar notch, and patellar sunrise views. Several different methods of imaging the patella tangentially (the sunrise view) have been described. Many of them carry eponyms, but there is minimal difference between the various views.

Ankle: A-P, lateral, and mortise (oblique) views.

Foot: A-P, lateral, and oblique. There are a number of special views of the foot which highlight various aspects of the skeleton. The three views just mentioned should be used to localize the injury, and target specific views. The Harris heel view allows examination of the calcaneus and subtalar joint in suspected calcaneal fractures.

Tomography

Tomography remains a useful tool in the imaging of the articular surfaces, such as the tibial plateau and the elbow. In addition, it can be used to image the cervicothoracic junction in the patient where it cannot be seen on plain film. Computed tomography has displaced much of the routine use of tomography, although its usefulness should not be overlooked. An accurate knowledge of the topographical anatomy is necessary for interpretation.

Computed Tomography

Computed tomography has revolutionized diagnostic imaging. The areas of greatest influence include the brain, spine, pelvis, and orthopaedic oncology. In the spine, visualization of degenerative disease as well as imaging of trauma has been improved. As a routine, all patients undergoing myelography have a CT scan performed after the dye injection. CT scans are performed on any spine trauma in which cord impingement is suspected. Additional software has been developed which allows the cross-sectional images to be reconstructed in orthogonal and nonorthogonal planes, as well as reconstructing three-dimensional models and films of the skeleton. Three-dimensional reconstructions are currently most often used in studying pelvic fractures.

In pelvic trauma, CT accurately assesses the congruity of the acetabulum. Bone fragments in the joint can be accurately identified. Three-dimensional reconstruction facilitates improved preoperative planning for reduction and fixation.

CT scans play a major role in the preoperative planning for tumor resection. The scan gives information about local extension as well as being a sensitive test for metastases (i.e., lung metastases in osteosarcoma). The scans also yield prognostic information as the tumor border can be visualized, and an initial assessment can be made about tumor aggressiveness.

Magnetic Resonance Imaging

Magnetic resonance imaging (MRI) is the newest modality available for the imaging of the musculoskeletal system. The major advantage of MRI is that it does not use radiation and thus can be safely used in pregnant women and young children. In addition, it is even better at imaging certain soft-tissue abnormalities than CT. Among its current orthopaedic uses are imaging of soft-tissue tumors, imaging of the spine, especially the intervertebral disc, and imaging of the cartilage and ligaments of the knee in suspected internal derangement of the knee.

Ultrasound

Ultrasound is commonly used in obstetrics, as a method of imaging the fetus without using radiation. Currently, its primary use in orthopaedics is imaging the rotator cuff and biceps tendon in shoulder problems, and evaluating a child's hip in suspected congenital dislocation. Although all of these problems can be imaged by arthrography, ultrasound is a noninvasive method with similar diagnostic potential.

Radionuclide Imaging

Radionuclide imaging, in the form of bone scans or skeletal scintigraphy, is used often in orthopaedics. The technique involves injection of a radioactive tracer into the blood, followed by imaging the entire body or parts of the body at set intervals to measure the uptake of the tracer. Several different techniques exist but the most commonly used tracer is a technetium compound ($^{99}Tc^m$), usually either a pertechnate or phosphate salt. Another commonly used tracer is gallium (^{67}Ga). Gallium is more costly and requires more radiation exposure but can be more sensitive in the diagnosis of osteomyelitis.

Bone scans are quite helpful in the diagnosis of osteomyelitis and stress fractures. Osteomyelitis may not demonstrate any plain film changes for up to two weeks but a bone scan will often show increased uptake in the first 2-3 days. Stress fractures that are undetectable on the plain radiograph can often be diagnosed by bone scan.

Bone scans are usually performed by injection of the tracer with a static phase whole body scan being performed approximately three hours later. Alternately, a three-phase bone scan can be performed, which is helpful in differentiating cellulitis from osteomyelitis. The three-phase bone scan consists of a localized static blood pool image immediately after injection, a dynamic flow curve performed immediately after injection (the radionuclide angiogram or the "poor man's arteriogram"), and a whole body static bone scan performed three hours after injection. Osteomyelitis will demonstrate increased uptake in both the late and immediate images, while cellulitis will usually show increased uptake only on the immediate images.

Bone scans are also helpful in the diagnosis and staging of bone and soft-tissue tumors. In this instance, the scan can show satellite or metastatic lesions as well as demonstrating evidence of bone invasion by a soft-tissue lesion.

Invasive Imaging

Several different methods of invasive imaging are useful in orthopaedics, notably arthrography, myelography, discography, and angiography.

Arthrography: Arthrography involves the injection of a radiopaque iodinated contrast material into a joint followed by plain radiographs of the joint. It is useful in multiple joint complaints, although its use in knee injuries has been largely supplanted by diagnostic arthroscopy. Arthrography is indicated to help diagnose a rotator cuff repair. Because of the lack of ossification of epiphyses, it is also useful in evaluating children's elbow and hip problems.

Myelography: Myelography involves injection of a radiopaque iodinated contrast material into the epidural space via a lumbar puncture. It is used to evaluate the spinal canal for the presence of disc pathology or possible intraspinal tumors. The procedure formerly carried a very high complication rate of postmyelogram headaches and nausea, but newer, water-soluble, nonionic, low-osmolality agents have lessened the incidence of these problems.

Discography: Discography consists of injecting a radiopaque iodinated contrast material directly into the nucleus pulposus, usually via a lateral approach. Plain radiographs of the discs are then performed. The procedure is performed for possible disc pathology, mostly degenerative disc disease. Although the appearance of the disc on radiograph is important, equally important is the amount of dye accepted by the disc, as degenerated discs will accept more. A normal lumbar disc accepts only 1.0 to 1.5 milliliters. Most important is the patient's response to the injection. When the injection exactly recreates the patient's typical back pain, this is presumptive evidence that the disc being injected is the source of the patient's pain.

Angiography: Angiography, primarily arteriography, has multiple uses in orthopaedics. It is used in trauma to evaluate the integrity of major arteries near the sites of fracture or puncture wounds. It is used in the workup of bone or soft-tissue tumors to determine the proximity of the major vessels and the resectability of lesions. The advent of CT and MRI has slightly decreased this indication; however, arteriography is now often used in orthopaedic oncology for evaluating the possibility of intraarterial injection of chemotherapeutic agents directly into a lesion. In addition, arteriography can be used to evaluate multiple vascular syndromes of the upper and lower extremities, including Raynaud's phenomenon, ulnar artery thrombosis, true and false aneurysms, and atherosclerotic disease.

Selected References

1. Ballinger PW. *Merrill's Atlas of Radiographic Positions and Radiologic Procedures.* 6th edition. 3 vols. St. Louis: C. V. Mosby, 1986.
2. Gehweiler JA, Osborne RL, Becker RF. *The Radiology of Vertebral Trauma.* Philadelphia: W. B. Saunders, 1980.
3. Putman CE, Ravin CE. *Textbook of Diagnostic Imaging.* 3 vols. Philadelphia: W. B. Saunders, 1988.
4. Resnick D. *Bone and Joint Imaging.* Philadelphia: W. B. Saunders, 1989.
5. Rogers LF. *Radiology of Skeletal Trauma.* 2 vols. New York: Churchill-Livingstone, 1982.
6. Sandler MP et al. *Correlative Imaging: Nuclear Medicine - Magnetic Resonance - Computed Tomography - Ultrasound.* Baltimore: Williams & Wilkins, 1989.

Chapter 5

Orthopaedic Emergencies and Emergency Room Techniques

Wounds, Open Fractures, and Open Dislocations

An open fracture is defined as one in which an open wound communicates directly with the fracture site or hematoma.[6] An open dislocation is one in which an open wound penetrates into the joint space and in which there is complete loss of congruity of the articular surfaces. Any open wound that communicates directly with a joint space, even if there has been no loss of congruity of the joint surfaces, must also be recognized.

All of these injuries are surgical emergencies. The potential for contamination and bone or joint sepsis is very high for two reasons: one, the obvious entry of contaminants through the open wound; and two, the great amount of stripping of soft tissues which necessarily occurs as a result of either an open fracture or dislocation. This second factor is clinically utilized to classify such fractures.

In an effort to prevent osteomyelitis or septic arthritis following open fractures or open joint injuries, these are considered to be surgical emergencies. The proper handling of these wounds in the emergency room is critical in the eventual success of any treatment. Definitive treatment requires knowledge of the classification of the wound as well as the fracture or dislocation.

Open fractures have been classified by Gustilo as described in Table 5-1:[7]

TABLE 5-1

OPEN FRACTURES

Grade I	-	An open fracture with a wound less than one centimeter in diameter.
Grade II	-	An open fracture with a wound greater than one centimeter in diameter, and less than 10 centimeters in diameter, but without extensive soft tissue loss or devitalization, and no vascular injury. This is a large category which some physicians define as any open fracture which is not a Type I or a Type III.
Grade III	-	An open fracture with a high-energy wound with extensive soft tissue loss or devitalization, or one in which there has been a major vascular injury.
Grade IIIA	-	A Type III injury, but one without extensive periosteal stripping or a vascular injury requiring repair.
Grade IIIB	-	A Type III injury accompanied by extensive periosteal stripping or gross contamination, such as in a farmyard injury.
Grade IIIC	-	A Type III injury accompanied by a major vascular injury requiring repair.

Open dislocations and open joint injuries can be considered similarly.

Definitive irrigation and debridement of open skeletal injuries in the emergency room is ill-advised. Some physicians may argue that Type I injuries could be handled in this manner. Yet precisely because it is the least contaminated, it should be handled the most sterilely, and these wounds must be treated in the operating room. In addition, the external appearance of the wound often bears no resemblance to the flora which will be found when examining the ends of the fracture site. The converse argument is that Type III wounds are so badly contaminated that they do not require perfectly sterile conditions. But iatrogenic introduction of contamination must be avoided, and these wounds are usually so extensive that debridement is usually not possible without appropriate surgical instruments and adequate lighting.

The management of open skeletal injuries begins, as always, with a history and physical examination. In the history, if the patient is able to give one, it is critical to document how long the wound has been open, the degree of contamination to which it may have been exposed (farmyard, factory, versus relatively clean home environment), and the status of the patient's tetanus immunization. Tetanus toxoid booster or tetanus immune globulin is given if indicated. (See Table 5-2 for recommendations about tetanus prophylaxis.)

TABLE 5-2

TETANUS PROPHYLAXIS

History of Tetanus Immunization	Tet-Prone Wound Td*	TIG*	Non Tet-Prone Wound Td	TIG
Uncertain	Yes	Yes	Yes	No
0-1	Yes	Yes	Yes	No
2	Yes	No+	Yes	No
3 or more	No#	No	No@	No

*	Td = Tetanus and diphtheria toxoids adsorbed (adult)
	TIG = Tetanus immune globulin (human)
+	Yes, if the wound is more than 24 hours old
#	Yes, if more than 5 years since the last booster
@	Yes, if more than 10 years since the last booster

(Reprinted with permission from *Guide to Antimicrobial Therapy 1989*, Jay P. Sanford, M.D., author and publisher. Reference: ACS Bulletin, 69: 22-23, 1984.)

Examination of the patient is obviously necessary to diagnose an open skeletal injury. Failure to notice an open wound communicating with a fracture can be of such disastrous consequences that all fractures should be considered open until proven otherwise. Since many of these injuries occur in the multiply traumatized patient, the orthopaedic examination is often given very low priority. The examiner must never fail to examine the posterior portion of the extremity or pelvis, as this is where most open fracture/dislocations will be missed. The axillae and groin areas must be inspected as an open wound may be concealed in these areas. If an extremity has an open wound and a fracture, it is an open fracture, until proven otherwise by direct probing of the wound. Since this procedure cannot always be done in the emergency room, these must be treated as open fractures in the operating room. In the emergency room it is important to evaluate and record the appearance of the wound, and the neurovascular status of the extremity.

Though some skeletal injuries are obvious by the physical examination, good radiographs are always necessary to plan proper treatment of the injury. However, in dealing with open fractures, priorities must be examined. The treatment of an open skeletal injury will almost always be initially concerned with treatment of the wound and secondarily with the fracture. It is inappropriate to send patients to the radiology department with known open wounds undressed and communicating with the open air with the intent of obtaining better x-rays to delineate the fracture.

All wounds should be initially dressed with soft, sterile gauze dressings, usually impregnated with Betadine, and covered by a nonconstrictive dressing, such as bias-cut stockinette. This type of dressing allows penetration of radiation sufficient to diagnose virtually all fractures.

If the patient has an obvious fracture, whether open or not, it should be splinted as soon as possible. If there is no neurovascular or soft tissue compromise, it is safest to splint the limb in the position in which it lies. However, if there is obvious gross deformity, gentle manipulation for anatomic positioning is usually recommended. Many emergency departments provide fenestrated aluminum extremity splints and these can be placed under the limb and held in place with loosely applied gauze rolls or bias-cut stockinette. If these are not available, a plaster splint can be made quickly.

Once a fracture is diagnosed, the extremity must be splinted as soon as possible, both to avoid further tissue damage, and to decrease the patient's suffering. In fractures diagnosed by examination, the splinting should be done prior to the patient being sent for radiography. Though the splint will slightly obscure bony details, for obvious fractures the radiographs will certainly be adequate for the initial study.

Once adequate radiographs have been obtained and an open fracture, dislocation, or intraarticular injury diagnosed, plans are made for definitive treatment in the operating room. The patient is prepared for surgery with an admission history and physical, laboratory studies, and the personnel in the operating suite and the anaesthesia department are notified.

The urgency of such problems is repeatedly emphasized to the emergency physicians and the operating room staff. It is well documented that the longer such injuries are exposed to air and potential contamination, the higher is the rate of infection.[14] Because of other injuries, or backlog in the operating room, it is not always possible to operate immediately on the patient with an open skeletal injury.

In these situations, a temporizing method of wound care is performed in the emergency room. The splints are removed and sterile dressings, which were applied earlier, are removed, and copious irrigation of all the open injuries in as sterile a manner as possible is performed. If a sterile jet-pulse irrigation system is available in the emergency room, it should be used if the patient is able to tolerate the discomfort. The wounds are redressed with sterile gauze and Betadine and the extremity resplinted. Prior to irrigation of the wound, a culture should be taken to allow accurate diagnosis of any bacterial contaminants.

Antibiotics are adiministered as soon as a diagnosis of an open skeletal injury has been made, whether by examination or by radiographs. A broad-spectrum cephalosporin is routinely given for open wounds. For Type III injuries or severely contaminated wounds, or in cases where there is a delay in going to the operating room, an appropriate dose of an aminoglycoside should be added. Even in cases where the patient has compromised renal function, it is usually safe to give one initial dose of the aminoglycoside. During the delay in going to surgery, the cephalosporin is administered on an appropriate schedule and, if there is no renal insufficiency, the aminoglycoside is added.

During any delay in going to surgery it is critical to reexamine the patient from time to time to assess the neurovascular status of the injury. Although this may have been intact at initial examination, since these are usually high-energy injuries, large amounts of soft tissue damage may have occurred. A neurovascular injury may not be apparent immediately but may subsequently develop. During the waiting period for surgery, the extremity should frequently be evaluated for the presence of a neurovascular injury or a developing compartment syndrome.

Compartment Syndromes

A compartment syndrome is defined as a condition in which the circulation and function of tissue within a closed space is compromised by increased pressure within that space.[9,10] The ultimate sequelae of an unrecognized or untreated compartment syndrome is often a functionless, useless distal extremity. Unfortunately, despite many advances in the diagnosis of the syndrome and in the awareness of it, this complication still occurs. It is critical that the physician always have a high index of suspicion to avoid potential disasters.

Compartments are defined as groups of muscle and neurovascular pedicles surrounded by an unyielding fibrous band. Multiple compartments have been defined, but clinically, those in the forearm and lower leg are of the most importance (Fig. 5-1). While compartment syndromes of the thigh and upper arm do occur, they are much less common. This is because the anatomy of the upper portion of the limbs yields more and allows more swelling before compartment pressure increases.

Compartment syndromes can occur after almost any musculoskeletal injury. They have been described after a single weightlifting workout, and chronic compartment syndromes in athletes are well known. Certain injuries, however, should immediately cause the physician to be suspicious of a possible compartment syndrome. Included in this are supracondylar elbow fractures in children, proximal and mid-shaft tibial fractures, electrical burns (especially in the forearm), and arterial or venous disruption. Unfortunately, compartment syndromes can also be caused iatrogenically by a dressing, splint, or cast which compromises circulation to a compartment.

The exact pathophysiology of a compartment syndrome is unclear. There are several popular conflicting hypotheses for the development of the syndrome. Early hypotheses considered arterial spasm to be important in the pathogenesis. More recently, Burton[2] and Ashford[1] suggested that small rises in pressure will often exceed a critical transmural pressure, causing many small vessels to close, resulting in cessation of flow. A third hypothesis considers a change in the arteriovenous (a-v) gradient to be the important factor. As small pressure increases occur within a compartment, venous pressure must increase to allow

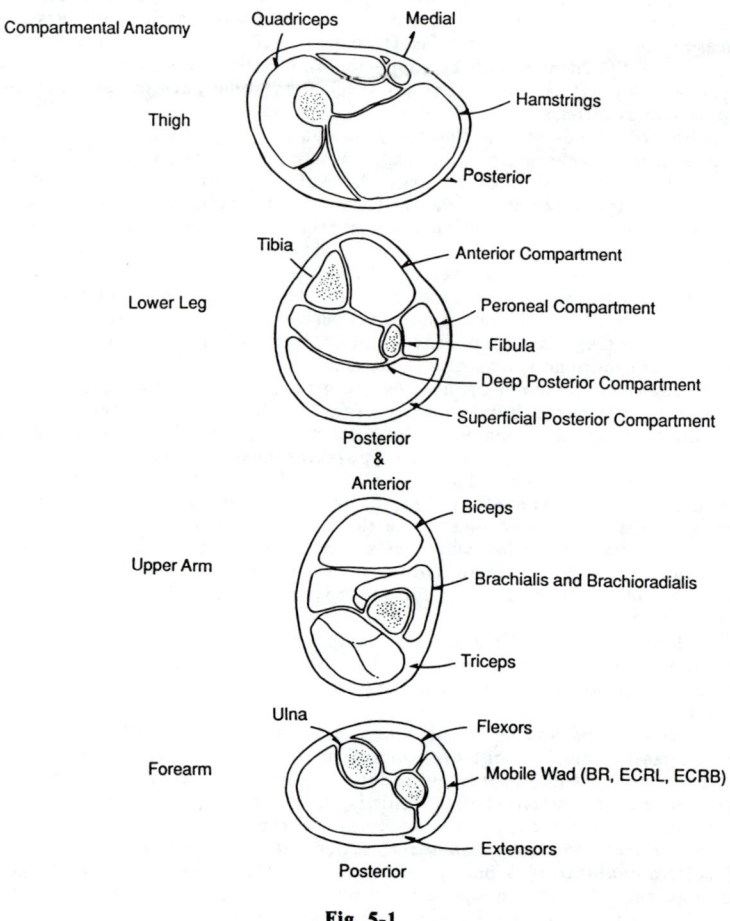

Fig. 5-1

Anatomy of the Compartments of the Thigh, Lower Leg, Upper Arm, and Forearm

venous flow to continue. If there is no change in mean arterial pressure this of necessity causes a decrease in the a-v gradient and a decrease in tissue perfusion. As pressure increases, the a-v gradient across the capillaries will eventually decrease to the point that flow is insufficient to perfuse the tissues at all.

All of the theories can be supported and criticized - both clinically and experimentally. It is likely that all three play some part in the developing compartment syndrome.

Regardless of the exact etiology, the danger of a compartment syndrome lies in permanent neuromuscular damage. Whether the damage occurs first to the nerves or the muscles is often argued. Actually, either answer is correct depending on the parameters. Paraesthesias and hypaesthesias in nerves can be seen clinically after only 30 minutes of ischemia, while muscle shows functional changes after 2-4 hours of ischemia time. However, permanent damage occurs first in muscle, at 4-12 hours, versus 12-24 hours for permanent nerve damage.[4] It is important to realize that permanent muscle damage may occur within four hours of untreated muscle ischemia. This period should be considered a critical limit for treating any suspected compartment syndrome. An impending compartment syndrome is a surgical emergency.

Today compartment syndromes are often diagnosed by measurement of compartment pressures, but for many years the diagnosis was made clinically. The clinical diagnosis is made on the basis of the four "P's" - pain (on passive motion), pallor, paraesthesias, and pulselessness. However the last "P," pulselessness, must be applied with cautious understanding of the syndrome. A distal pulse may be audible, palpable, or even strong in the presence of an existing compartment syndrome, since the compartment pressure may be severe enough to cause muscle ischemia yet not occlude the major artery(ies) in the compartment. If the clinician awaits pulselessness to diagnose a compartment syndrome, the muscle and nerve damage may be severe and catastrophic at this stage.

Three additional "P's" may assist in making the diagnosis: paralysis, purple color, and point (loss of two-point discrimination). The latter may be the earliest sign of an impending compartment syndrome and the former two are definitely late signs.

The sine qua non of the diagnosis of a compartment syndrome rests upon pain on passive motion, out of proportion to the anticipated pathology. In addition, the limb will be firm and indurated and palpation of the compartments often will cause excruciating pain. This is, unfortunately, a subjective evaluation which requires some experience to diagnose accurately. In children or the multiply injured, not fully responsive, patient, it is not very reliable. It is also difficult to evaluate in a patient after he has taken large doses of analgesics. Similar to the situation in which pain medicine is denied the patient with an acute abdomen, it must be dispensed with caution in a patient with a possible compartment syndrome.

Although pallor will develop in an extremity with increased compartment pressures, it occurs secondarily. Actually, the limb will first become cyanotic (purple - "P") because of increased venous congestion secondary to the increased compartment pressure. Unfortunately, neither may be present so this sign is neither necessary nor sufficient to diagnose the syndrome.

Paraesthesias will always develop, eventually, in a compartment syndrome, but one should never wait for their development. Recovery of function occurs in only 13% of patients who had some motor loss at the time of diagnosis.

Certain compartment syndromes are obvious to a physician with experience in diagnosing the syndrome. In these cases, clinical judgment is often sufficient cause to take the patient to the operating room for fasciotomies to relieve compartment pressures. In those cases where it is not an obvious diagnosis, the measurement of compartment pressures is often beneficial.

There are several well-known methods of measuring compartment pressures, notably the Whitesides technique, the wick catheter method, and the slit catheter method. The wick or slit catheter is thought to be slightly more accurate but requires a more elaborate setup. In addition to accuracy, these methods have the ability to continuously monitor the pressure over several hours or even days. In addition, commercial compartment monitors are now available. These are certainly the easiest to use, but their reliability has not yet been proven clinically.

When measuring pressures is thought to be necessary, it is imperative that all compartments have their pressures measured. In the forearm this includes the anterior and posterior compartments, as well as the mobile wad of Henry (brachioradialis, extensor carpi radialis brevis and longus). In the lower leg, four compartments are measured: the anterior, peroneal or lateral, superficial posterior, and deep posterior (Fig. 5-1).

It is unclear what pressure exactly defines a compartment syndrome. Normal compartment pressure in an uninjured extremity is probably zero or close to it. Measurements of under 30 torricelli can safely be observed, but it is important to observe them with either serial measurements or clinical observation. Some physicians consider 40 torricelli a critical number and will operate on these extremities to release the pressure. A measurement between 30 and 40 torricelli makes the decision to treat or not to treat difficult and depends on the clinical situation, including the duration of the elevated pressure, and experience of the examining physician.

In addition, it is becoming increasingly clear that the reading of the compartment pressure is related to the patient's systemic blood pressure. Compare two patients - one in hypovolemic shock with a mean arterial pressure of 50 mm Hg, and a compartment pressure of 30, while the second is a hypertensive patient with a mean arterial pressure of 110 mm Hg and a compartment pressure of 40 torricelli. It seems obvious that the first patient is at higher risk to experience compartment damage from lack of perfusion because of the gradient present in the compartment. The patient's systemic blood pressure should never be neglected when considering the compartment pressures. Whitesides has mentioned 30 mm Hg below the patient's diastolic pressure as a critical compartment pressure. Based on our clinical experience, we consider one compartment pressure reading over 40 torricelli or serial readings over 30 torricelli (over 8-12 hours) to be an indication for immediate fasciotomy.

Surgical treatment of compartment syndromes consists of a skin incision, followed by fasciotomy of all involved compartments. Details can be found in the standard surgical texts. Important considerations here, however, are that the fascia is <u>never</u> closed, and that the skin is often left open. Skin closure will either be by delayed primary closure or by a skin graft of some type.

Should surgical treatment not be elected, it is difficult to say if any specific conservative treatment is indicated. Although some people advocate elevation of the extremity to increase venous return and decrease the arterio-venous (a-v) gradient, most experts on this problem condemn this. Elevation of the limb, by aiding venous return and decreasing the a-v gradient, may prevent the development of a syndrome when pressures are normal. But once a compartment syndrome (i.e., elevated compartment pressure) is diagnosed, elevation of the limb should be avoided. This is because the venous pressure cannot be lowered below the compartment pressure, and elevation of the limb will decrease the arterial pressure head, thereby lowering the a-v gradient.

Iatrogenic compartment syndromes must be treated promptly by release of the offending dressing or cast. It is difficult to make the diagnosis when an extremity is circumferentially enclosed by the dressing. When there is the slightest suspicion of a compartment syndrome, the clinician must release the dressing and examine the limb. It is important to fully release the dressing or cast. If the cast is split, the underlying cast padding <u>must</u> also be split, to the depth of the skin, as it can be a very tight, constrictive dressing.

Injuries Compromising Neurovasculature or Soft Tissues

The first consideration in any injury to an extremity should not be the obvious injury, but the neurovascular status of the injured limb. This should also be carefully documented in the medical record.

Many musculoskeletal injuries present with compromised neurovasculature. It is not always possible to tell immediately if there has been transsection of a major vessel or nerve, or if the compromise is simply a matter of arterial spasm or neuropraxia.

The physician's dictum "Do not make the patient worse," must therefore be a primary consideration. If there is not transsection of a vessel or nerve, manipulation of a fractured or dislocated extremity runs the risk of iatrogenic transsection. If the extremity is grossly displaced or dislocated, <u>gentle</u> manipulation is appropriate to diminish pain, relieve vasospasm, and allow easier splinting. If there is any question of causing neurovascular injury, the extremity should be splinted as is and reduction performed in the operating room. In that case, reduction under direct vision or in a more controlled environment will minimize the risk of neurovascular damage.

Where there may be neurovascular compromise but the patient will be treated without operative intervention, the problem then becomes one of experience. Orthopaedic or trauma residents in their early training period or medical students should never reduce these injuries without first discussing them with their chief resident or a member of the attending staff. In matters of possible vascular damage, the question becomes one of reduction before undergoing arteriogram, if it is indicated. It is a difficult decision which should be made by someone with experience in these injuries.

Where there is obviously neurovascular compromise because of a displaced fracture, the neurovascular status of the extremity must take priority. The fracture should be grossly reduced by distal distraction as well as possible and as soon as possible - even before sending the patient for radiographs. In general, this problem occurs most commonly with severely displaced ankle fractures presenting with either a pulseless or hypaesthetic foot.

The same problem occurs where skin is tented and at risk for necrosis by a displaced fracture or dislocation. If neurovascular status is intact, reduction of a badly displaced fracture may entrap nerves or vessels and create more damage. Such a problem again requires experience and judgment as to when and the method which will be used to reduce the injury.

No patient should remain in the emergency room with an obvious fracture and with the extremity not splinted. Besides avoiding any further soft tissue damage, it is far more humane as it reduces motion at the fracture site and thus reduces the patient's pain. In such cases, even before being seen by the orthopaedist, the emergency room physician should have the extremity splinted, elevated slightly, and probably have an icebag applied to the area of the injury to diminish soft-tissue swelling.

Several good ready-made splints are available. Many emergency crews splint extremities with air splints. If other splints are available, we would recommend these be removed on arrival at the emergency room. Air splints make examination of neurovascular status impossible; they are so bulky that radiographs in more than one projection are difficult to obtain; and if inflated to too high a pressure, they can cause a compartment syndrome and neurovascular damage. If no other ready-made splints are available in the emergency room, a padded plaster splint should be carefully applied to the limb. When in doubt, "splint them where they lie" and obtain consultation from a physician of more experience and judgment.

Complete and Partial Amputations

Complete or partial amputation of an extremity or a digit is common, especially in industrial areas. With today's modern microsurgical techniques, many of these can be successfully replanted and become functional limbs and digits. However, proper management of the extremity and digit is essential to optimize chances for a successful replantation.

In complete amputations, there are basically two methods of preserving the amputated part: 1) wrapping the part in a cloth moistened with saline or lactated Ringer's solution, and placing the bundle in a plastic bag to be placed on ice; or

2) immersing the part in saline or lactated Ringer's solution in a plastic bag, and then placing the bag on ice.

When a patient arrives in the emergency room shortly after such a problem, without referral, it is important that one of the above methods be used to store the amputated part. If an outside physician calls and refers such a problem to you, clear and concise instructions about management of the amputated part should be given.

We prefer the immersion method for several reasons: 1) the part is less likely to become frostbitten; 2) the part is less likely to be strangled by the wrapping; 3) the instructions are more easily understood by the primary care physician; and 4) maceration secondary to immersion is not a problem.[15]

In partial amputations, it is important to maintain all connections between the parts. Even a small dorsal skin bridge on a digit may contain important venous channels and improve the chance of replantation. It is therefore important to handle the proximal and distal portions very carefully when examining the patient.

In these cases a small, fairly loose, gauze dressing is applied after the initial examination. An icebag is then placed over the dressing. The layer directly apposed to the injury should be slightly damp. A gauze sponge soaked in Betadine and fully wrung out makes a good bottom layer. This type of dressing serves several purposes: 1) the Betadine gives some antibacterial protection; 2) the loose dressing prevents strangulation of the extremity or digit; 3) the damp under-layer prevents desiccation of parts while awaiting transport to the operating room; 4) a loose, small dressing initially applied allows easy reexamination by the attending surgeon upon his/her arrival, and minimizes the chance of further damage by unwrapping a tight, bulky dressing; and 5) the icebag cools the amputated part and diminishes its metabolic requirements, allowing more time for repair.

The proximal portion of the extremity or digit also demands attention. In cases of an amputated or partially amputated arm or leg, where life-threatening hemorrhage is occurring, it may be necessary to clamp major bleeders. Obviously, here the patient's life becomes the primary consideration. In general, however, bleeding from the proximal extremity should be handled with pressure and a dressing which is reinforced as necessary. Clamping bleeders in the emergency room, when not necessary, damages an unknown amount of vascular intima which may compromise vascular repair. Also, in the ER, where exposure is usually less than optimal, one may cause damage to other vital structures (nerves, tendons) by blindly clamping bleeders. It should be reserved for life-threatening situations, usually proximally in a limb.

Prompt preparation of the patient for transport to the operating room is critical, especially when a patient has been referred from a distance. Tissues will survive for about 4-6 hours if not cooled (warm-ischemia time), while with proper cooling, they may survive up to 12-24 hours (cold-ischemia time). The muscle, as in a compartment syndrome, suffers permanent damage first, and thus, digits may survive even longer (up to 30 hours), as they have little or no muscle tissue.

Unstable Spine Management

Although orthopaedic surgeons rarely deal directly with life-threatening injuries, they frequently manage situations of almost equal importance - an unstable or potentially unstable spine, with the patient's future neurologic status at risk. Rarely are such patients seen by the orthopaedist immediately at the scene of the injury. A few guidelines for management at the scene are in order, however, as they are also applicable in the emergency room for the patient who was improperly handled at the scene of injury.

Any patient sustaining an injury above the clavicle or a head injury resulting in an unconscious state should be suspected of having an associated cervical spine injury. Such patients should not be moved until an ambulance and the emergency medical technicians (EMTs) arrive at the scene. This caution is advised because they have the equipment needed to safely move the patient. Once the priorities of respiratory and cardiovascular stabilization have been managed, the immobilization of the patient in a neutral supine position becomes paramount.

When the proper equipment has arrived, the patient should not be moved until his cervical spine is immobilized in a firm plastic orthosis (Philadelphia or Malibu collar). While one person then places axial distraction on the head, these cervical orthoses, which are comprised of two sections, can be slipped under the neck without moving it. The patient can then be safely moved onto a firm spine board. The injury victim should never be lifted, but moved only in a log-rolling-type manner, in which his thoracic and lumbar spines are not flexed or rotated. After the patient is moved onto the spinal board, sandbags should be placed tightly against the sides of his/her neck and head, and the head should be secured to the board by taping across the forehead and circumferentially around the board. In addition, the patient's torso should be secured to the board by a seat-belt-type arrangement. At any time after this initial evaluation, should the patient need to be moved, he/she must be moved in the same manner until adequate radiographs have been obtained to completely exclude a spinal injury.

In certain cases, the semirigid plastic cervical collar should not be used.[15] This is true, for example, whenever it is suspected that the patient has suffered an injury to a great vessel or to the trachea. The collar would then act as a tourniquet, constricting an injured, swelling neck, and hiding from view an expanding hematoma or subcutaneous emphysema. In these cases, it is imperative that sandbags and circumferential tape be used to secure the victim's head. The patient can still be moved onto a spine board, but his cervical spine should be protected. A safe method in this situation is for the physician to place both his palms under the patient's scapulae, on opposite sides of the neck, and approximate both of his elbows closely together while bracing them against his abdomen. The patient's head is held by the mover's forearms while the patient is moved the few inches onto the spine board.

Once the patient with a spinal cord injury has arrived in the emergency room, management follows that standard for a trauma victim.[3] Attention is first directed to the airway, breathing, and circulation (ABC). If a patient with a potential cervical spine injury requires intubation, this should be done with the patient's neck stabilized in one of the above-mentioned semirigid collars. Nasotracheal intubation is preferable to orotracheal in these cases as the spine needs to be moved less. If there is any difficulty intubating in this manner, and the situation demands immediate airway control, one should proceed immediately either to emergency tracheostomy or cricothyroidotomy.

Examination of the patient proceeds with a thorough and accurate neurologic evaluation, with emphasis on noting the level of any neurologic deficit. Once a level of deficit has been established, it is especially important to accurately document it carefully as well as any sparing which occurs below this level. Patients with any degree of sparing of motor, sensory, or reflex function below their level of injury, have a good prognosis for neurologic improvement.[15] Patients whose neurologic injury is immediate and complete rarely recover any neurologic function below the level of injury.

It is not always possible on initial evaluation to document neurologic sparing, but this should not rule it out. After spinal injury, many patients will be in spinal shock, which may mask some remaining functions. Exams should be repeated over the first 24-48 hours to look carefully for any returning function, indicating both an incomplete lesion and the resolution of spinal shock. Often used for this are the anal wink and bulbocavernosus reflex (see the section on physical examination). However, most authors feel that motor or sensory sparing provides the best basis for prognosis, as opposed to reflex sparing.

Halo Collar Placement and Management

Today, the standard of care for unstable cervical spine injuries is use of the halo collar with either traction or a jacket to immobilize the neck. First introduced in 1959 by Perry and Nickel,[12] the halo has virtually replaced the older systems of Crutchfield, Gardner-Wells, and Vinke tongs for traction. While those systems provided adequate traction, they could not immobilize the spine in more than one plane.

The injuries which require halo traction and jacket can best be found by referring to the standard references. Once it is determined that a patient will need the halo, the physician should proceed immediately with its application. Most major hospitals today provide a "halo tray" which sterilely provides everything necessary to place the halo.

A reliable system for placement of the halo collar should consist of: 1) back panel; 2) occipital support to hold the head; 3) interconnected antero-posterior and mediolateral bars; 4) halo attachment casting; and 5) four positioning knobs to provide head and halo ring adjustment in all planes (Fig. 5-2).[8]

Placement begins by positioning the patient (still on the spine board and still with semirigid collar in place) at the end of the bed so that his head overhangs the bed. The head must be stabilized manually with axial distraction during this maneuveur. While one doctor continues to stabilize the spine, the back panel is slid under the patient's back between the scapulae in direct line with his neck. The occipital support, is then attached to the back panel and tightly secured. The patient's head may then be supported by the occipital support although it is preferable to have one assistant loosely support the patient's head throughout. The semirigid collar should be maintained in place throughout for assurance.

Once the head is supported by the occipital panel, the appropriate size halo ring is selected. It is placed in the approximate position desired, and secured to the occipital support by means of the halo attachment casting (Fig. 5-2). By use of the adjustment knobs and anteroposterior and mediolateral bars, the halo can then be accurately held in position until it is placed exactly as desired. The halo is then swung away from the skull and the skin sterilely prepared and shaved. It is usually a simple matter to return the halo to the predetermined position, as long as it is moved in only one plane.

Optimum positioning of the halo is critical to ensure stability, durability and patient comfort. Four holes are placed in the scalp, two anteriorly and two posteriorly. The front holes are centered in the groove at the upper margin of the eyebrows - between the supraciliary ridge and the frontal prominences. Posteriorly, the halo is placed about 1/4" above the ears. This placement of the halo ensures that it will be below the maximum diameter of the skull and thus will not migrate superiorly.[11]

Sagitally, the front pins should be placed just superior to the outer half of the eyebrows, to avoid the supraorbital nerve and vessels. They should be placed as close to the midline of the eyebrow as possible, as the thickest mass of bone is central. Some surgeons place the pins lateral to the eyebrows under the hairline, to avoid all scarring. This position may cause three problems, 1) since the pin penetrates the temporalis muscle, chewing causes tethering of the muscle by the pin and is usually very uncomfortable; 2) the temporal bone is quite thin in this region and pin penetration or loosening may occur; and 3) since the posterior pins are placed opposite the anterior pins, this lateral position causes the posterior pins to be very close to the anterior pins, and multiplane stability is decreased.[11]

Once the pin positions have been selected, and the skin has been sterilely prepared, the pins are inserted. Each pin should placed until they just touch the skin. One front pin and the diagonally opposite back pin are tightened to maximum finger tension. The other pair is likewise tightened. A torque screwdriver is then used to tighten the pins, again tightening them in pairs first.

Optimum tightness of the halo pins has been shown to be 6 kg-cm.[11] This cannot always be achieved initially but the closest torque below this amount to which all pins can be tightened should be chosen. Unequal tensions should not be used as the halo will migrate in the direction of the pin of least tension.

Daily pin care is instituted, which consists of sterilely cleaning the pin sites daily. To be certain of adequate purchase, the pins should be carefully

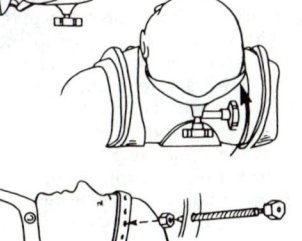

(1)

(2)

(3)

(4)

(5)

Fig. 5-2

Placement of the Halo Collar and Jacket

In (1) and (2) the head of the patient is stabilized by an assistant while the jacket is placed on the patient. In (3) the head support is placed under the mattress of the bed and under the patient's head. Alternately, (3) may be performed before (1) and (2) to better stabilize the head. In (4) the head support is used to position the patient's head in preparation for placement of the halo ring. In (5) the halo ring is positioned about the patient's head and four halo pins are inserted as described in the text. After placement of the pins and the halo ring, the halo ring is attached to the jacket by means of struts, which are held to the halo ring by nuts.

tightened daily for three days, and then checked for tightness every three days three more times. After this initial pin care, they need be tightened or checked only every two weeks. They should be maintained at the optimum 6 kg-cm torque, but slightly less torque may have to be accepted. Pins should not be routinely tightened more than a full turn at any visit. This may indicate a loose pin which has migrated into the skull's inner table. If such a pin has a torque far less than the optimum, it should be removed and a new one placed. In that case, the diagonally opposite pin must also be replaced.

Often the halo collar is initially placed to a cervical traction device set up at the head of the bed. The halo collar comes with an excellent traction device for easy attachment. The exact positioning of the neck will depend on the type of injury. The amount of traction needed for reduction of a cervical fracture or dislocation can be estimated as ten pounds to distract the head and five pounds for each interspace. Thus a C_{4-5} fracture-dislocation would probably require thirty pounds of traction. We usually start out with less than this, perhaps 20, and take serial radiographs to evaluate the reduction. It is imperative that STAT portable lateral C-spine radiographs be taken after placement of the unstable cervical spine into traction. It is equally imperative that this roentgenogram be viewed as quickly as possible. Based on the initial radiographs, adjustments in the traction can be made as needed.

Once the reduction is adequate in traction, the patient is usually placed in a halo jacket for long-term care. The plastic jackets have front and back shells which are connected by the halo bars and Velcro straps. In addition, the front shell has a foldback front piece which allows sternal compression in the event of life-threatening cardio-respiratory problems.

The patient can be fitted for the jacket as soon as it becomes obvious that he will need prolonged halo immobilization. Proper placement of a halo jacket requires at least two, and preferably three people. The jacket shells are placed into position by sliding the back shell under the patient and placing the front shell on him. The patient is then carefully brought upright with his neck supported throughout the maneuver. The head is centered such that the ears are directly over the top of acromia, when viewing the patient laterally. In an A-P direction the head and neck should be aligned to look directly forward, with no lateral tilt or rotation. The neck is left in approximately the position it was in while in traction, and the halo bars and pins are all securely tightened. An immediate lateral C-spine radiograph is ordered and checked quickly. Adjustments can be made as needed.

In young children and infants, halo jackets are often not available in proper sizes. In these situations, the halo collar, and over-the-shoulder halo bars, are held in place with a Minerva jacket - a jacket made of plaster which is placed over the shoulders and around the upper torso.

Placement of Traction Pins

This section will describe only skeletal traction, as the other types of traction are outlined in the section specifically devoted to traction. It is now unusual to select pure skeletal traction as the treatment of choice for a fracture, but it is often used as a temporizing measure. There are many instances where skeletal traction may have to be applied in the emergency room.

By far the four most common sites of placement for traction pins are: 1) proximal tibia; 2) distal femur; 3) olecranon; and 4) calcaneus. We will outline the basic method of placement and the anatomic landmarks for placement in these four sites.

A serious complication of a skeletal pin is a pin tract infection and consequent osteomyelitis. Therefore, the entire area around the insertion site should be thoroughly prepped and draped as if for a full surgical procedure. After choosing the entry and exit sites, both areas are then infiltrated with a local anaesthetic. A small skin incision is made over the entry site. The appropriate Steinmann pin or Kirschner-wire is placed in a hand drill and pushed through the soft tissues of the incision until it contacts bone. The pin is then "walked up" and down the bone to estimate the exact position to penetrate the bone. The pin is drilled through the bone, and after it exits the opposite cortex, the pin will tent the skin. Another small incision is made directly over the area of tenting to allow the pin to exit the skin. The pin should be placed so that equal lengths protrude from the skin on both sides of the extremity. Many times the pin will exert undue pressure over the skin incisions in a transverse plane. When this occurs, extend the skin incisions by making them into cruciate incisions. The pins can then be trimmed to a length adequate to hold the traction bow or K-wire tractor. Usually, Betadine-soaked gauze is placed around the pin at the skin sites, and cork knobs are placed on the ends of the pin for protection.

Placement is carefully chosen to avoid damage to neurovascular structures. The pins should be placed perpendicular to the long axis of the bone, except the femoral pin (see below), and they should be parallel to the sagittal plane of the body.

Proximal tibia pins are placed more often than others. These should be inserted from the lateral side to avoid damage to the peroneal nerve on exiting the skin. The landmark is to place the pin one-to-two fingerbreadths below the tibial tuberosity in the midportion of the tibia (Fig. 5-3). Putting the pin more proximal places it through too much cancellous bone, which is weaker. Placing it more distal, while in stronger cortical bone, risks damage to the peroneal nerve as it moves anterior after it passes around the fibular neck.

Distal femoral pins are inserted from the medial side to avoid damage to the femoral artery on exiting the skin. The entry site is the adductor tubercle (Fig. 5-3). In very large people, this can be difficult to palpate but it is just proximal to the medial epicondyle which usually can be felt. Placing the pin distally risks entering the intercondylar notch, while more proximal placement risks damaging the femoral artery near Hunter's canal. The pin should not be

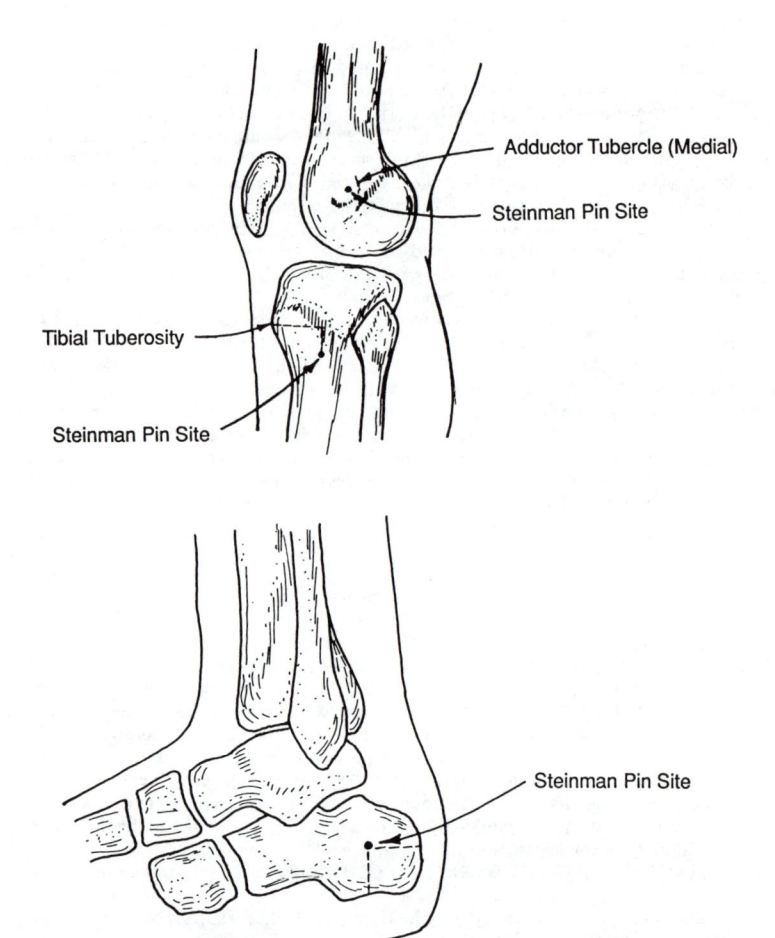

Fig. 5-3

**Steinman Pin Insertion Sites in the Distal Femur,
Proximal Tibia, and Calcaneus**

placed perpendicular to the femoral shaft because this would angle the pin distally as it exits. Place this pin perpendicular to the knee joint.

Olecranon pins are placed from the medial (ulnar) side to avoid damaging the ulnar nerve. The nerve should be palpated with one hand to keep its position in mind throughout. With the elbow in 90 degrees flexion, the end of the olecranon is palpated. The entry site is 1 1/2" from the distal end of the olecranon. The olecranon is not very thick so care should be taken to try to enter its midsubstance directly. This is done as noted above by walking up and down the bone with the pin after entering the soft tissues.

To avoid problems with the ulnar nerve, a small screw-hook may be inserted directly into the proximal end of the olecranon. This is placed in line with the longitudinal axis of the ulna with the elbow flexed 90 degrees. Traction is necessarily then of the overhead type.

Calcaneal pins are placed from the medial side to avoid damage to the posterior tibial neurovascular pedicle. The posterior tibial pulse should be palpated with one hand during the initial placement. The entry side is 1" above the plantar border of the calcaneus and 1" anterior to the dorsal border. Alternately, this can be described as 1" posterior and 1" inferior to the medial malleolus. The exit should be chosen so that the pin is perpendicular to the tibia. Ideally, it will not exit too close to the fibula, as this can again damage the peroneal tendons, as well as the sural nerve, lesser saphenous vein, and peroneal artery (Fig. 5-3).

Joint Aspiration

In the emergency room, it is often necessary to aspirate joints for diagnostic purposes, especially to rule out a septic joint. Occasionally, however, joint aspiration is used to evacuate a hematoma to give the patient pain relief, or to inject a local anaesthetic or steroid. Whatever the reason for aspiration, it is necessary to know how to enter the joint to perform the aspiration.

The main complication of joint aspiration is introducing infection into a sterile joint. This is a disaster and should be kept in mind throughout. The most important principle of joint aspiration is to use strictest sterile technique. The basic principles of joint aspiration are as follows:[13]

1) **MAINTAIN STRICT STERILE TECHNIQUE.** This is too important not to repeat.

2) Enlarge the joint space by positioning. This also stretches the joint capsule and facilitates entry into the joint by the needle.

3) Use bony landmarks. These are more reliable than soft tissue landmarks.

4) Select sites that avoid neurovascular structures and do minimal damage to tendons.

5) Avoid scoring articular cartilage by probing blindly for the joint.

6) Do not inject into vessels. Avoid this by always aspirating before injecting anything.

The landmarks for joint aspiration require a good knowledge of anatomy. Many of these landmarks have been modified in recent years because of the expanding use of arthroscopy of joints other than the knee.

Finger Joints: Palpate the joint dorsally with the finger in slight flexion. After the joint has been located, extend the digit and enter dorsolaterally or dorsomedially, volar to the extensor mechanism. This method also avoids injecting the neurovascular structures to the fingers as they are just volar to the mid-sagittal plane of the digits.

Wrist Joint: This joint is entered dorsally. If there is any difficulty in entering the wrist joint, the hand can be suspended in Chinese finger traps to help open the joint space. There are two main entry sites, called the 3-4 and 4-5 sites by Watanabe[16] in his book on arthroscopy. The 3-4 site is most often chosen and enters the wrist between the 3rd and 4th extensor compartment (compartment 3 contains the EPL, and compartment 4 contains the EDC and EIP). This is far easier to identify than the 4-5 site, as one can palpate Lister's tubercle on the distal radius and enter the skin just distal to this, volar-flexing the wrist to facilitate entry. The 4-5 site is between the 4th and 5th extensor compartment (compartment 5 contains the EDQ). This is used when one is concerned about ulnar-carpal pathology, but other than palpating the distal ulnar, there is not a good bony landmark to identify the entry site (Fig. 5-4). Other options for entry are 6R and 6U, i.e., 6R is radial to the ECU and 6U is ulnar or volar to the ECU.

Elbow Joint: The elbow can be entered either ulnarly or radially, but the radial approach is preferred because damage to the ulnar nerve is not uncommon using an ulnar approach. While the radial approach can damage the radial nerve, the nerve is anterior to the humerus at the elbow and further from the entry site.

The elbow should be flexed 90 degrees. Rotatory positioning of the hand is not important, for this will be controlled during landmark identification. Palpate the lateral humeral epicondyle. With another finger of the same hand, palpate the radial head just distal to epicondyle. To be certain you have identified the radial head (which is deep to some fairly thick muscles) pronate and supinate the forearm and feel the radial head rotate. The entry site is now between the two palpating fingers (Fig. 5-5).

Shoulder Joint: Anterior approaches to the shoulder are described but are not generally recommended. The posterior approach gives easy access to the glenohumeral joint and avoids the risk of damaging the brachial plexus or cephalic vein. In addition, the posterior approach finds the joint more superficial.

The patient should be seated and the entire shoulder, both anterior and posterior, should be prepped and draped. Palpate the most lateral edge of the acromion process. Choose an entry site one cm medial and one cm distal to this. With the other hand, palpate the coracoid process anteriorly. Now aim the needle for the coracoid process and it should enter the joint. A spinal needle should be used, as the joint is deep, especially in muscular or obese individuals.

Subacromial Bursa: With the patient seated, palpate the lateral portion of the acromion process. Enter the skin at this point. Have the needle strike the

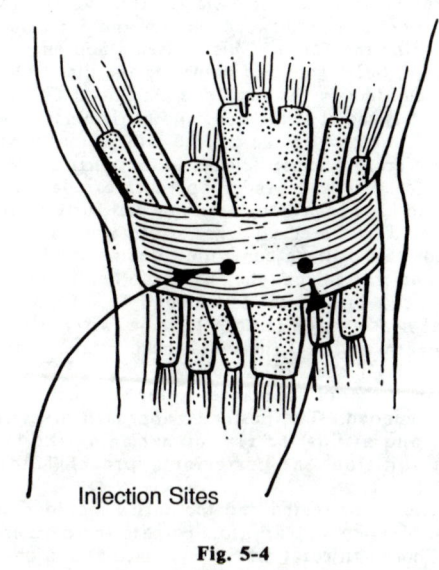

Injection Sites

Fig. 5-4

**The 3-4 (left) and 4-5 (right) Portals for
Aspiration of the Wrist Joint**

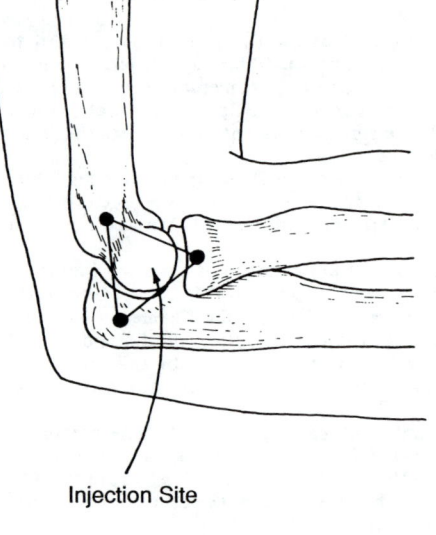

Injection Site

Fig. 5-5

The Site for Aspiration of the Elbow Joint
The triangle's landmarks correspond to the lateral epicondyle,
the radial head, and the olecranon.

acromion and then "walk" the needle down the acromion and push it in further when it easily passes under the acromion. It is then in the subacromial bursa.

Acromioclavicular joint: This is very superficial and can be palpated. Enter from a superior approach. To ease identification of the joint, have the patient forward flex his arm to 90 degrees. The joint will then be readily felt if either the examiner or the patient adduct and abduct the arm.

Toe Joints: Use a dorsal approach and enter beneath the extensor mechanism as described for finger joints.

Ankle Joint: Two approaches can be used, either medial or lateral. With either approach, entry is just anterior to the corresponding malleolus. Entry is facilitated by plantarflexion of the ankle. Palpate the joint while dorsi- and plantarflexing the ankle to aid identification of the joint. The ankle joint is notoriously difficult to enter.

Knee Joint: Multiple approaches can be used, as has been shown arthroscopically. This is the largest joint in the body and the easiest to enter. Either a medial or lateral approach is fine, but a medial approach is probably easier with the knee in extension as the patella can be rocked up anteriorly to aid in entry.

If the patient will allow the knee to be flexed to 45 degrees, do so. Palpate the inferomedial and inferolateral borders of the patella, and enter the knee through either portal, going just medial or lateral to the patellar ligament.

With the knee in extension, palpate the tibial plateau and slightly sublux the patella towards the side you are entering. Enter the joint just above the tibial plateau going under the patella.

Hip Joint: This is a difficult joint to enter and should probably be done only by or in the presence of someone experienced in the approach. Several approaches have actually been described, but the medial approach is the most universal.

Palpate the femoral pulse just as it exits the inguinal ligament. The entry site is 1" lateral to the femoral pulse at this point. Going lateral 1" will also make the entry site approximately 1" below the ligament. Needle entry is then straight down (perpendicular to the coronal plane of the body). A long spinal needle is used, but usually the joint is easily entered by this approach. If any difficulty is obtained with this approach, fluoroscopic guidance is recommended for hip aspiration (Fig. 5-6).

The lateral approach can also be used. The greater trochanter is palpated and the needle inserted just superior to it. The needle is directed 45 degrees cephalad, and parallel to the table (patient supine). The femoral neck will usually be met and the needle can then be directed slightly cephalad and proximal to enter the iliofemoral joint.

Proficiency in entering the various joints of the body is gained only by experience. Useful aids in joint aspiration include: 1) studying the anatomy of a skeleton prior to aspiration; 2) injecting sterile saline or lactated Ringers' solution into the joint and observing its easy exit through the needle hub as the joint fluid adds viscosity to the solution; 3) rotation of the joint (especially the femoral and radial heads) to detect motion or "scraping;" and 4) fluoroscopic assistance in complex or difficult situations.

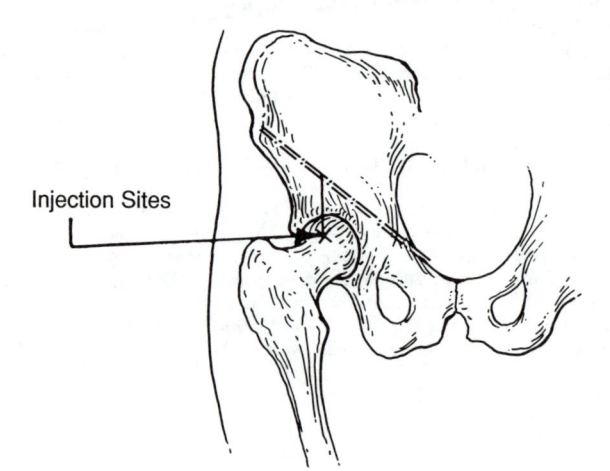

Injection Sites

Fig. 5-6

Injection Site for Aspirating the Hip Joint

References

1. Ashton H. The effect of increased tissue pressure on blood flow. **CORR.** 113: 15-26, 1975.
2. Burton AC. On the physical equilibrium of small blood vessels. **Am. J. Physiol.** 164: 319-329, 1951.
3. Committee on Trauma, American College of Surgeons. Advanced Trauma Life Support Course. American College of Surgeons, 1984.
4. Evarts CMcC and Mayer PJ. Complications: Compartment syndromes. In: *Fractures in Adults*, Rockwood CA, and Green, DP (eds.) Philadelphia: J. B. Lippincott, 1984.
5. Green BA et al. Acute spinal cord injury: current concepts. **CORR.** 154: 125-135, 1981.
6. Gregory CF. Open fractures, In: *Fractures in Adults*, Rockwood CA and Green DP (eds.) Philadelphia: J. B. Lippincott, 1984.

7. Gustilo RB and Anderson JT. Prevention of infection in the treatment of one thousand and twenty-five open fractures of long bones. **JBJS.** 58A: 453, 1976.

8. Hardaker WT, Reed WO, Vaughn DW, and Clippinger FW. Duke Halo-Positioner, improved technique for halo application. **Ortho. Review.** 8(10): 566, 1984.

9. Matsen FA. *Compartmental Syndromes.* New York: Grune & Stratton, 1980.

10. Mubarak SJ and Hargens AR. *Compartment Syndromes and Volkmann's Contracture.* Philadelphia: W. B. Saunders, 1981.

11. Perry JL. The halo in spinal abnormalities. **Ortho. Clin. North Am.** 3(1): 69-80, 1972.

12. Perry JL and Nickel VI. Total cervical-spine fusion for neck paralysis. **JBJS.** 41A: 37, 1959.

13. Pruce AM, Miller JA, and Berger IR. Anatomic landmarks in joint paracentesis. **Clin. Symposia.** Vol. 10, No. 1, Jan-Feb 1958.

14. Ritmann WW, Schibli M, Matter P, and Allgoewer M. Open fractures - long-term results in 200 consecutive cases. **CORR.** 138: 132-140, 1979.

15. Urbaniak JR. Replantation: Preparation of the amputated part. In: Green DP. *Operative Hand Surgery.* New York: Churchill Livingstone, 1982.

16. Watanabe M. *Arthroscopy of Small Joints.* Tokyo: Igaku-Shoin, 1985.

Chapter 6

Fractures, Dislocations, and Other Musculoskeletal Injuries

The Language of Fractures

As with all branches of medicine, fractures are discussed in a language peculiar to the specialty involved. It is imperative that the physician or medical student learn this language in order to accurately describe a fracture to the senior resident or attending physician. Without such an accurate description, effective communication about treatment modalities is not possible.

Fractures are classified according to: 1) the bone involved; 2) the location of the fracture; 3) the pattern of the fracture fragments; and 4) the amount of anatomic disruption. Following are the four main locations in which a fracture can occur:

Fracture Location

Diaphysis: The diaphysis is the main shaft of long, tubular bones (Fig. 6-1).

Metaphysis: The metaphysis is the flared end of a long bone, and is located between the diaphysis and the physis (Fig. 6-1).

Physis: The physis is present only in a growing bone. It is the cartilaginous growth plate which occurs near the end of a long bone. At skeletal

81

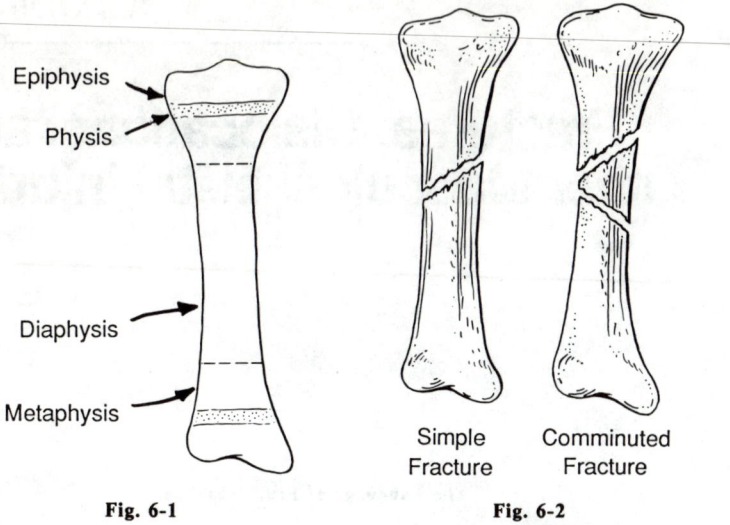

Epiphysis

Physis

Diaphysis

Metaphysis

Fig. 6-1

**The Four Main Parts
of a Long Bone**

Simple
Fracture

Comminuted
Fracture

Fig. 6-2

**Simple and Comminuted
Fractures**

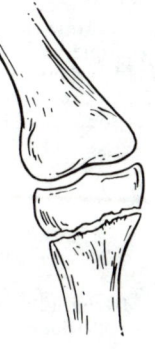

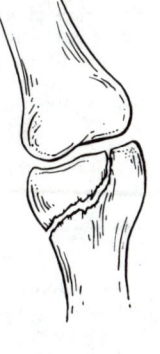

Extra-Articular
Fracture

Intra-Articular
Fracture

Fig. 6-3

Extra- and Intraarticular Fracture Patterns

maturity, the physis ossifies and fuses with the epiphysis and the metaphysis (Fig. 6-1).

Epiphysis: The epiphysis is the end of a long bone between the physeal cartilage and the articular cartilage (Fig. 6-1).

Fracture Patterns

Closed Fracture: A closed fracture is one in which the skin is intact overlying the fracture and its hematoma.

Open Fracture: An open fracture is one in which there is a break in the integument which communicates with the fracture site or fracture hematoma. The size of the break in the integument is immaterial in classification as an open fracture, although it carries prognostic significance. See Table 5-1 and the section on Open Fractures in Chapter Five (*Orthopaedic Emergencies and Emergency Room Techniques*) for a discussion of the prognostic significance.

Simple Fracture: A simple fracture is one in which there is a single fracture line such that the bone is divided into only two separate fragments (Fig. 6-2).

Comminuted Fracture: A comminuted fracture is one in which the bone is divided into more than two fragments by the fracture lines. There are sub-classifications of comminuted long bone fractures but it is important to remember that a fracture with 100 fragments, and one with two large fragments and a smaller one - are both considered comminuted. However, there is a difference in prognostic significance (Fig. 6-2).

Extraarticular Fracture: An extraarticular fracture is one in which the fracture line does not enter a joint cavity (Fig. 6-3).

Intraarticular Fracture: An intraarticular fracture is one in which the fracture line enters a joint cavity (Fig. 6-3).

Transverse Fracture: A transverse fracture is one in which the fracture line is perpendicular to the long axis of the involved bone (Fig. 6-4).

Oblique Fracture: An oblique fracture is one in which the fracture line subtends an oblique angle with the long axis of the involved bone (Fig. 6-4).

Spiral Fracture: A spiral fracture is an extreme case of an oblique fracture in which the plane of the fracture through the bone rotates about the long axis of the bone (Fig. 6-4).

Longitudinal Fracture: A longitudinal fracture is parallel to, or nearly parallel to, the long axis of the involved bone (Fig. 6-4).

Impacted Fracture: An impacted fracture is one due to a compressive force which causes the end of a bone to be driven into the contiguous metaphyseal region of the bone without displacement. It may, however, be angulated or rotated (Fig. 6-4).

Pathologic Fracture: A pathologic fracture is a fracture through abnormal bone.

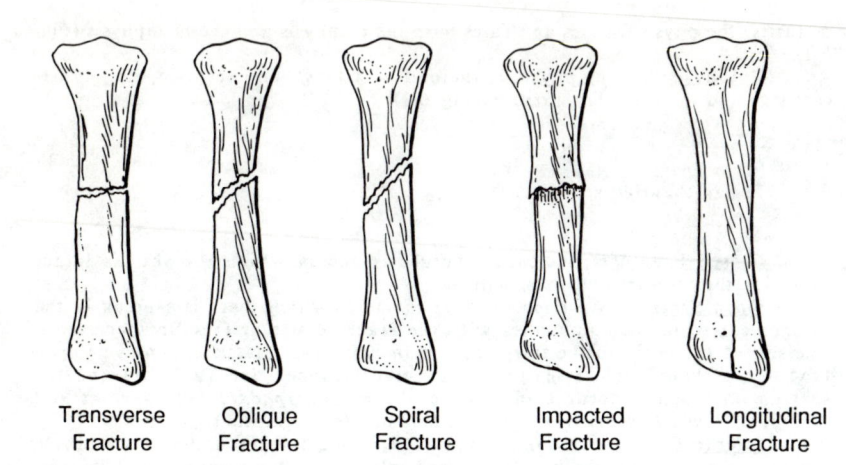

| Transverse Fracture | Oblique Fracture | Spiral Fracture | Impacted Fracture | Longitudinal Fracture |

Fig. 6-4

The Five Main Directions of Fracture Patterns

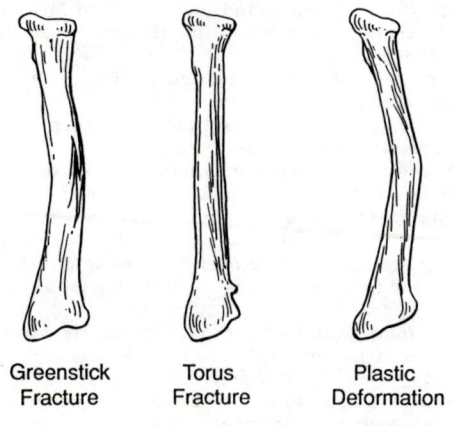

| Greenstick Fracture | Torus Fracture | Plastic Deformation |

Fig. 6-5

Special Fracture Patterns Seen in Children

Stress (or Fatigue) Fracture: Considered by some to be a type of pathologic fracture, this is a fracture through normal bone that has been subjected to cyclic loading at loads which, acting singly, are not sufficient to cause an acute fracture.

Greenstick Fracture: A greenstick fracture is an incomplete fracture in which only one cortex is broken while the opposite cortex and periosteum remain intact. It is much more common in children (Fig. 6-5).

Torus Fracture: A torus fracture is also more common in children. It is an impaction injury in which the cortex of a long bone buckles with no loss of cortical continuity (Fig. 6-5).

Plastic Deformation: Plastic deformation is exclusively an injury occurring in children's bones. It occurs when a child's bones simply bend with no break in either cortex. This is because children's bones are more porous and consequently, less brittle (Fig. 6-5).

Physeal Injury: This is an injury through the physeal plate in a developing child. These injuries have their own system of description and are discussed in more detail below.

Dislocation: Dislocation is technically defined as total loss of congruity between the articular surfaces of a joint. Anything less than total loss of congruity should be strictly termed a subluxation. However, extreme subluxations are often termed dislocations, but this is not technically correct.

In addition to describing the location of the fracture and the pattern of the fracture lines and fragments, it is necessary to be able to describe the degree of anatomic disruption. Loss of normal anatomy can occur because of displacement, angulation, rotation, and separation.

Anatomic Disruption

Displacement: This is a measure of the translational distance between the corresponding cortices of the fracture fragments. An example can be seen in Fig. 6-6 (left). The tibia has two fracture fragments. The distal fragment has moved with no angular change in the longitudinal axis of the fragment. It has been translated laterally.

Angulation: Angulation measures the angle between the longitudinal axes of the main fracture fragments (Fig. 6-6 [middle]). Here the two tibial fragments are angulated and lines are drawn through each fragment corresponding to their longitudinal axis. These lines intersect with an angle of 20 degrees, which is the measure of the angulation of the fracture. It is important to be able to describe the direction of angulation, and this can cause difficulty. The reason is that different texts describe angulation in different methods.

In Figure 6-6 the tibial fragments are angulated such that the distal end of the distal fragment points laterally. Although it would be proper to say that the

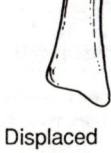
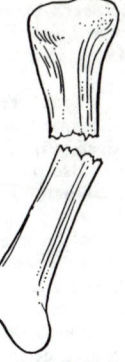
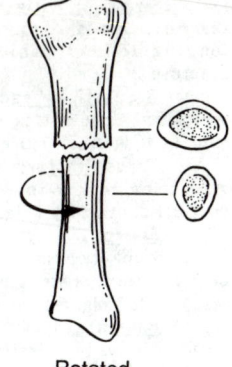

| Displaced | Angulated | Rotated |
| Fracture | Fracture | Fracture |

Fig. 6-6

Fracture Displacement, Angulation, and Rotation

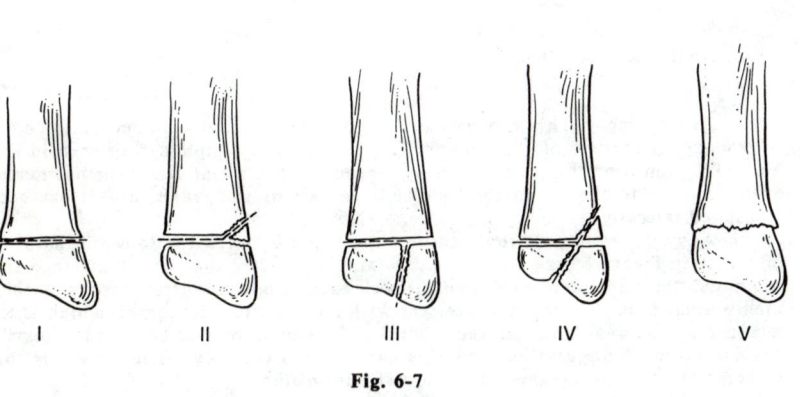

    I   II   III   IV   V

Fig. 6-7

Salter-Harris Classification

fracture is angulated into valgus (distal fragment directed laterally), there is no similar analogy to describe anterior-posterior angulation. Some authors describe this fracture as angulated laterally, meaning that the distal fragment is directed laterally, while others would call this medial angulation, meaning that the apex of the fracture is directed medially. For consistency, we recommend describing the direction of the apex of an angulated fracture (e.g., apex medial, apex dorsal, etc.).

It is best to simply describe the fracture pattern and not attempt what may be an ambiguous short-cut in terminology. In Figure 6-6, if you say, "It is angulated with the apex directed laterally," there is less chance for misinterpretation.

Rotation: Rotation is a twisting about the longitudinal axis of one of the fracture fragments. It is the most difficult type of fracture disruption to see on radiographs and it is also the deformity which remodels the least as the fracture heals. Rotation can be evaluated better clinically than it can be radiographically. One clue to rotatory deformity can be seen in Fig. 6-6 (right). Here the fracture is not angulated or displaced, but the apparent diameter of the bone changes on opposite sides of the fracture line.

Separation: Separation describes the situation in which there is a gap between the fracture fragments.

It is now possible to fully describe an adult fracture. When calling a senior resident or attending physician to describe an injury, a complete description might be as follows, "The fracture is a closed, simple, transverse, extraarticular fracture of the distal radial metaphysis. The distal fragment is displaced dorsally one centimeter, and the fracture is angulated 20 degrees with the apex directed volarly." The common eponym of this fracture is a Colles' fracture, but the above description conveys much more information.

Physeal Injuries

Children's fractures can be more difficult to describe accurately because of the presence of the growth plate. There are several classification systems for fractures involving the physis. By far the most widely used is the Salter-Harris system, which is as follows:

Salter-Harris Type I: In this injury the fracture line goes directly through the physis. There may be a slight gap between the fragments but since the physis is not radiopaque, the gap can usually only be appreciated by a comparison film of the opposite extremity. The diagnosis is often a clinical one and immobilization and non-weightbearing until the child is symptomatically better are usually sufficient (Fig. 6-7).

Salter-Harris Type II: In this injury, the fracture line is mostly through the physis, but it exits one cortex such that a small fragment of metaphysis is included with the fracture fragment containing the physis and epiphysis (Fig. 6-7).

Salter-Harris Type III: In this injury, the fracture line is mostly through the physis, but it exits one cortex such that a small fragment of epiphysis is included with the fracture fragment containing the metaphysis and diaphysis (Fig. 6-7).

Salter-Harris Type IV: In this injury, a fracture line crosses the physis such that both fracture fragments contain portions of the metaphysis, physis, and epiphysis (Fig. 6-7).

Salter-Harris Type V: In this injury, there is no definite fracture line, and like the Salter-Harris Type I, this injury cannot be easily diagnosed radiographically. The injury involves a crush injury to the physis in which the metaphysis and epiphysis are acutely impacted upon one another. Unfortunately, the diagnosis is often a retrospective one and this injury carries a very high risk of growth plate arrest (Fig. 6-7).

The Salter-Harris classification is an excellent system in that it conveys prognostic information about each injury. As one goes from a Type I to a Type V, there is a greatly increased risk of growth arrest or deformity of the growth plate. There have been descriptions of a few, very rare, injuries to the growth plate which some authors term Types VI or VII. In addition, the above classification has been broken down further by Ogden. However, the above five categories are sufficient for most pediatric physeal injuries.

Radiology of Fractures

While it might seem a simple matter to diagnose a fracture from a radiograph, certain points can be made. **If a fracture is diagnosed, it is imperative to evaluate the joints proximal and distal to the fracture with radiographs.** Many concurrent fractures and dislocations have been missed because this rule was not followed. While it can be argued that a good exam of those joints will determine the need for a radiograph, many times the patient will be in too much pain to allow a good exam, and it is safer to simply radiograph the adjacent joints.

There are standard views that radiologic technicians use for each joint, usually beginning with an AP (anteroposterior) and lateral view. Often the physician will desire additional views. The standard views and certain special views are discussed in Chapter Four (*Radiologic Evaluation of the Orthopaedic Patient*). In addition, certain special views will also be mentioned below in discussing the individual fracture types.

Basic Fracture Biomechanics[1]

Fractures occur due to four main types of forces acting on bones - tension, compression, bending, and torsion.[1] It is important to understand the difference in the forces because they cause characteristic fracture patterns, especially in long bones. Often, it is possible to deduce the force causing the fracture by analyzing the fracture pattern. This information can then be used to aid in reducing a fracture by reversing the force that caused it.

Tension: Tension is a force applied to a bone or a portion of the bone such that the portion under tension is increasing in length.

Compression: Compression is a force applied to a bone or a portion of the bone such that the portion under compression is decreasing in length.

Bending: Bending forces can be termed either pure two-point bending or three-point bending forces. In pure bending, forces are applied to opposite ends of a bone in the same direction. In three-point bending, two forces are applied as in pure bending and a third force is applied between the other two but in the opposite direction (Fig. 6-8).

Torsion: Torsion is a force applied that causes a bone to rotate about its long axis.

One must remember that the above forces rarely occur in isolation. Specifically, when a bone is subjected to three-point bending forces, the cortex from which two forces are applied will be in tension and the opposite cortex will be under compression (Fig. 6-9).

The characteristic patterns produced by the four main forces are as follows:[1]

TENSION: The fracture pattern is straight transverse. Usually tension occurs only about a portion of the bone. Pure tension applied to a bone is extremely rare.

COMPRESSION: Compression causes an oblique fracture pattern. If there are no other forces involved, the oblique fracture will subtend an angle of 45 degrees with the long axis of the bone.

BENDING: As mentioned, bending causes one cortex to be under tension and one cortex to be under compression. Consequently, the fracture pattern will be a combination of the two patterns. The fracture pattern will be mostly transverse (along the tension side) but will propagate obliquely on the compression surface.

TORSION: The fracture pattern will be a spiral or long oblique type.

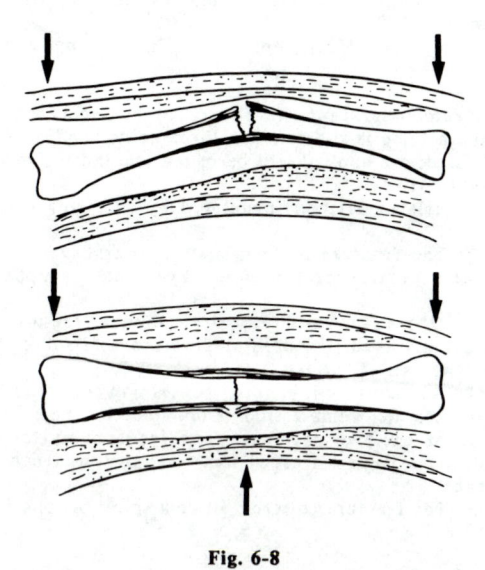

Fig. 6-8

**Examples of a Poorly Applied Cast (top) and a
Properly Applied Cast (bottom) [see text]
Cast at bottom shows the use of three-point bending applied against a soft-tissue
hinge.**

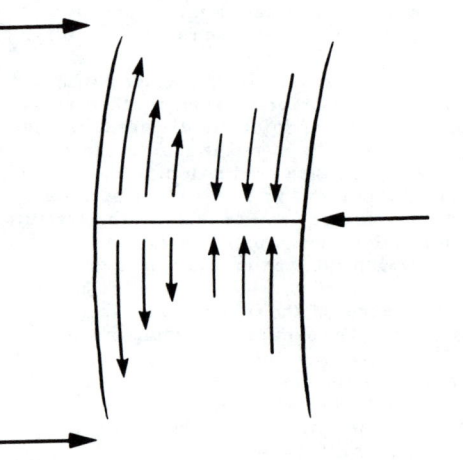

Fig. 6-9

The Three-Point Bending Principle
The side on which two forces are applied is under tension,
while the opposite cortex is under compression.

Closed Reduction - Basic Techniques[3]

After having evaluated the fracture pattern carefully, and deciding if it can be treated by closed reduction and immobilization, it is necessary to know how to do this. Every fracture is different, and the exact technique of reduction depends on the individual fracture. However, there are well-established principles that should guide the practitioners in reducing fractures and dislocations, provided he/she is supervised in his/her initial attempts.

First, by studying the fracture pattern and applying the biomechanical principles mentioned above, one should be able to deduce the mechanism of injury which caused the fracture. Secondly, it must be realized that stability of a fracture, after reduction, depends on the fracture pattern to a degree, but also depends a great deal on the soft tissue envelope surrounding the fracture. Simply stated, closed reduction of fractures involves reversing the original injury mechanism and holding the fracture by using the cast or bandage to apply proper pressure to the soft tissue envelope.

Reduction of the fracture actually is a bit more difficult than simply reversing the mechanism of injury. In Fig. 6-10 (top), an example of a fracture is shown and the fracture site shows that the ends of a fracture are never purely linear but rather have multiple areas of interdigitations. Attempting to merely reverse the fracture will cause these bone shards to impinge on one another and prevent reduction.

Impaction of the fragments on one another during reduction is prevented by first longitudinally distracting the fracture fragments, then gently exaggerating the mechanism of injury to disengage the ends of the fracture. Reduction is then performed by reversing the mechanism. The best example of such a reduction is shown in the closed manipulation of a Colles' fracture shown in Fig. 6-10. Here the physician's hands are placed on opposite ends of the fracture site, with the thumbs gently palpating the fracture ends opposite the apex of the fracture. Both hands pull longitudinally in opposite directions to distract the fracture (Fig. 6-10), then the fracture angulation is slightly increased, and finally, the fracture is reduced by reversing the mechanism, pushing volarly with both thumbs at the ends of the fracture fragments.

Several points must be followed concerning this basic method of reduction: 1) the three steps (distraction, exaggerate mechanism, reverse mechanism) should be done in one smooth, continuous motion; 2) it usually requires more force than one might imagine; and 3) pain will cause muscle spasm, and reduction will not be possible without adequate anesthesia in the form of a hematoma block, digital block, axillary block, intravenous Xylocaine (Bier block), or some other appropriate form of analgesia.

Further elaboration concerning the soft tissues is necessary. Commonly, attention is directed only to the bones, as they are so vividly seen on radiographs. But it cannot be overemphasized that the reduction is maintained using the soft tissue hinge. This soft-tissue hinge is illustrated in Fig. 6-11. Most long-bone fractures will have a hinge of soft tissue (most importantly, the periosteum) on

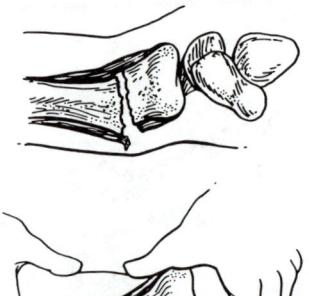

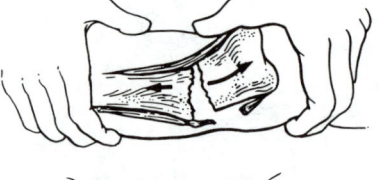

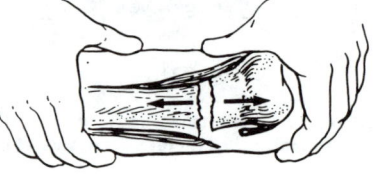

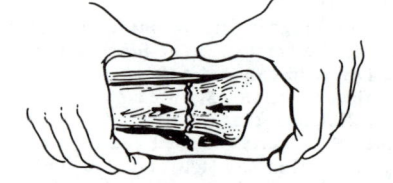

Fig. 6-10

The Basic Steps in Fracture Reduction [see text]

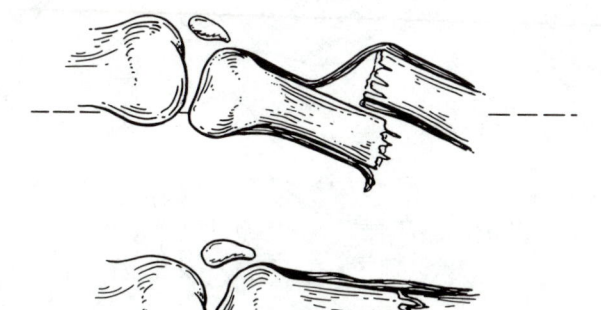

Fig. 6-11

**Fractured Tibia with an Intact Soft-Tissue Hinge on the Anterior Surface (top)
This is used to maintain fracture reduction (bottom).**

one cortex of the fracture. Usually, the hinge overlies the cortex opposite the apex of an angulated fracture.

When a soft-tissue hinge exists on one cortex of a fracture, it is almost impossible to overreduce the fracture. The hinge will remain intact and prevent this. However, the fracture can redisplace if the soft tissues are not used properly to maintain the reduction. Maintenance of the reduction is performed by applying a cast or splint such that the principle of three-point bending is used. Fig. 6-8 shows examples of properly (bottom) and improperly (top) applied casts.

The first cast shown (Fig. 6-8 [top]) fits the limb well but does not apply pressure properly against the soft-tissue hinge. Therefore, nothing is holding the fracture stable, as the soft tissue is loose and the fracture can displace. In the second example (Fig. 6-8 [bottom]), the cast is bent against the cylinder of the leg and illustrates the principle of three-point bending. The ends of the cast provide a force against the same cortex which contains the soft-tissue hinge. The middle of the cast pushes against the fracture site at its apex such that the soft-tissue hinge is maintained under tension. This will prevent the fracture from re-displacing and although the cast does not look as elegant to the uninitiated, it is an excellent cast. Charnley has stated, "Curved plaster makes straight bones."[3]

Should one place the dressing before or after reducing the fracture? It depends on the amount of help available, the fracture pattern, and the practitioner's experience. Charnley recommends applying a few layers of plaster, reducing the fracture in the wet cast, and then finishing the cast.[3] This requires excellent and quick casting ability, and the ability to reduce the fracture quickly. To do this, there should be minimal swelling so that the fracture ends can be felt through the early layers of plaster. In lieu of applying plaster first, it is helpful to have an assistant maintain the reduction while the practitioner applies the cast or splint. While learning to reduce fractures, it is probably better to reduce the fracture and then apply the cast or splint; in fact, we routinely prefer this sequence.

Special Fractures - Pathologic and Stress

As mentioned above, a pathologic fracture is a fracture through abnormal bone. A stress (or fatigue) fracture is a fracture through normal bone, but one that has been subjected to cyclic overloading at loads normally not sufficient to cause a fracture. A pathologic fracture does not have to occur through a tumor in the bone. In fact, the most common cause of pathologic fractures is osteoporosis.

It is important to always recognize pathologic fractures. While certain radiographs will show an unmistakable lesion in the area of the fracture, it is critical that a high index of suspicion be maintained for those fractures occurring with minimal trauma in seemingly healthy patients. This should always arouse suspicion of a pathologic fracture.

In cases of bone tumors, treatment of the fracture depends on establishing the correct diagnosis. Occasionally, the radiographic appearance is pathognomonic and biopsy is not necessary. Radiographic diagnosis of bone tumors is aided by evaluating four aspects of the lesion: 1) the margins of the lesion; 2) the periosteal reaction to the lesion; 3) the matrix pattern of the lesion; and 4) the location of the lesion.[15]

The margins of a bone tumor are classified as either a geographic pattern, a moth-eaten pattern, or a permeative pattern. Examples of each are shown in Fig. 6-12. A geographic pattern, especially one with thick, sclerotic borders, suggests a slow-growing benign process which allows the bone time to wall off the lesion. Both moth-eaten and permeative patterns suggest a more aggressive lesion and can be suggestive of a malignancy.[15]

The periosteum can react to a bone lesion in several manners, which are shown in Fig. 6-13. Generally, more benign lesions cause less reaction, which is usually manifested as a thickening or very slight elevation. More aggressive

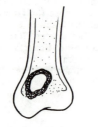

Geographic   Moth-Eaten   Permeative

Fig. 6-12

Patterns of Bone Destruction by Tumors

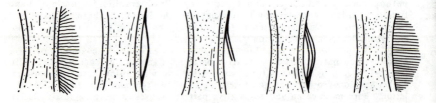

Fig. 6-13

Types of Periosteal Elevation

lesions cause ominous-appearing periosteal reactions such as the sunburst pattern, spiculated pattern, onion-skinning, or Codman's triangle.[15]

The matrix of a bone lesion can be either osseous, cartilaginous, fibrous, combinations of the above, or there can be no matrix, as in a simple cyst. Osseous matrices produce a typical blastic appearance on radiographs. Cartilaginous matrices are radiographically characterized by either a stippled or flocculated pattern, often described as "C's and O's" or an "alphabet-soup" appearance. Fibrous matrices appear radiographically as a hazy, soft density, often termed a ground-glass appearance.[15]

The location of the lesion in the bone is of critical importance. Most bone lesions occur in the metaphysis because that is the area of most active growth of the bone. The only two lesions which commonly occur in the epiphysis are chondroblastomas (Codman's tumor), and giant-cell tumors. Chondroblastomas occur only in the epiphysis. Diaphyseal lesions are typically small round-cell tumors, such as Ewing's sarcoma, multiple myeloma, and lymphoma of bone, or metastases.

Finally, the above information must be interpreted in light of the patient's age, as different neoplasms are more common in different age groups. For example, in patients over 60 years old, it should be remembered that the most common cause of a bone lesion is a metastasis. Several of the references list the most common bone tumors and their age distributions in large series.[5,13,25] By using this information, and the above four radiographic parameters, it is often possible to be quite specific about the differential diagnosis of a bone lesion.

Frequently, the radiograph will be equivocal. Additional staging studies such as computed tomography, magnetic resonance imaging, bone scans, and arteriograms may better define the lesion, but often open or needle biopsy is necessary to establish the diagnosis. Biopsy of a bone lesion should not be undertaken lightly. Enneking has stressed that it is often more difficult to plan and perform the biopsy than it is to do the definitive operation. Because the incision and biopsy will contaminate all the intervening tissue planes, it must be planned carefully so that all contaminated tissue can be removed during the definitive procedure.[9]

All staging studies should be done prior to performing a biopsy.[9] This is because bone tumors often bleed profusely and are difficult to control, even during biopsy. Performing the biopsy will often spread hematoma around the area of the tumor and make interpretation of the imaging studies almost impossible.

Further discussion of the details of biopsy and definitive tumor surgery is beyond the scope of this monograph. Interested readers are referred to Enneking's text for further study.[9]

Stress Fractures

The treatment of stress fractures depends on the bone involved and the activity which caused the stress fracture. The classic stress fracture is a "march" fracture - the stress fracture of the second metatarsal shaft suffered by Army recruits on long marches. Other common sites are the tibial shaft (runners), and the tarsal navicular (basketball players).

In all cases, treatment of the stress fracture should include removing the offending activity causing cyclic overload. For the above fractures, this includes an appropriate length cast (below-knee for the foot fractures and above-knee for the tibial fracture) and non-weightbearing as an activity. After the fracture is healed, the patients need to be advised about resuming the activity more gradually or in some way altering their biomechanics or environment to decrease the overloading.

Basics of Fracture Management

Fractures may be treated by either closed or open methods. There are advantages and disadvantages to both methods, and there are also specific indications and contraindications for the use of both methods.

The advantage of open reduction is that it is often possible to achieve anatomic alignment of a fracture, and to rigidly stabilize it using internal fixation. If rigidly stabilized, it is often possible to begin weightbearing and/or early motion of adjacent joints. This prevents what the AO/ASIF group (Arbeitsgemeinschaft fuer Osteosynthesfragen/Association for the Study of Internal Fixation) calls "fracture disease."[20] Fracture disease includes all the complications of immobilization and recumbency, including muscle atrophy, soft tissue atrophy, loss of joint motion, joint contractures, decreased articular cartilage viability, and increased risk of pulmonary and thromboembolic complications.

The primary disadvantage of open reduction is that a closed fracture is converted to an open fracture, with the attendant higher risk of infection. In addition, surgical exposure causes disruption of the surrounding soft tissues and circulation, which may compromise healing of the fracture. Also, the scarring of surgery may later interfere with muscle function and limit motion in the adjacent joints.

The main advantage of closed reduction and immobilization is that a closed fracture remains closed, with no increased risk of infection. In addition, other complications of surgery are not risked, and usually the hospital stay is shorter (if needed at all), and the cost of treatment is generally less.

The main disadvantage to closed treatment of fractures is that it is almost impossible to achieve exact anatomic reduction, and external stabilization by casts and splints can never be as rigid as properly applied internal fixation. In addition, casts and splints must often immobilize adjacent joints to be effective, and this can cause problems with loss of joint motion, especially in the elderly. Finally, in intraarticular fractures, the inability to achieve exact anatomic alignment predisposes to future problems with degenerative arthritis.

Absolute indications for open reduction are as follows:[4]

1) Fractures irreducible by manipulation or closed means.

2) Displaced intraarticular fractures, where the fragments are sufficiently large to allow internal fixation.

3) Certain displaced physeal injuries - mainly displaced Salter III and IV injuries.

4) Major avulsion fractures with significant disruption of an important muscle or ligament. Included in this group are fractures of the greater tuberosity of the humerus, the greater trochanter, the olecranon, the patella, the intercondylar eminence of the tibia, and the tibial tubercle.

5) Nonunion of a fracture which has received adequate treatment by a closed method.

6) Replantations of extremities or digits. In this case, rigid fixation is necessary to protect the repair of the neurovascular structures.

Relative indications for open reduction are as follows:[4]

1) Multiple fractures. Although individual fractures may be treated acceptably by closed methods, the multitrauma patient with multiple fractures is often better treated by open reduction/internal fixation (ORIF) of most of his/her major fractures. This allows early mobilization of the patient and helps prevent the complications of fracture disease.

2) Loss of reduction following closed methods.

3) Fractures accompanied by neurovascular disruption. Because the soft-tissue envelope remains intact this is not an absolute indication, as in replantation. However, stabilization of such fractures will allow better protection of the neurovascular repair.

4) Pathologic fractures. ORIF of pathologic fractures is a more humane treatment when these fractures are quite painful.

5) Delayed union of a fracture which has received adequate treatment by a closed method.

6) Avoidance of the morbidity and mortality associated with recumbency and immobilization. This is especially true in brain-injured patients or the elderly, and allows for easier nursing care.

7) Fractures for which closed treatments are known to be ineffective. Fractures in this category would include femoral neck fractures, Galeazzi fractures, both-bones forearm fractures in adults, and Monteggia fractures. See the discussion of specific fracture groups in the following section.

Relative contraindications to open reduction are as follows:[4]

1) An active infection or osteomyelitis is often felt to be an absolute contraindication to the implantation of a foreign body in the form of an internal fixation device. However, recent investigations suggest that even infected fractures will heal better when rigidly stabilized if the infection can be kept under control until the fracture is healed.[10] At that point the device can then be removed, and the problem changes from one of treating an infected nonunion (a very difficult problem) to one of treating osteomyelitis (a merely difficult problem).

2) Severely comminuted fractures or fractures where the fragments are too small to accept placement of internal fixation devices.

3) Bone that is too osteoporotic to allow secure internal fixation.

4) Abnormal skin conditions or surrounding soft tissues which might greatly increase the risk of infection.

5) General medical problems which contraindicate the use of anaesthesia.

6) Nondisplaced, stable fractures which are not at risk to displace or angulate with weightbearing or early motion.

Specific Fractures/Dislocations

The following discussion concerns the most common types of skeletal injuries. It is not intended to be encyclopaedic. Emphasis will be placed on radiologic evaluation, classification schemes, the basics of treatment, and the most common complications. The decision of whether to treat open or closed is critical and will be discussed in some detail, although open methods of treatment will be mentioned only briefly. All fractures are assumed to be closed initially. Treatment of open fractures begins with debridement of the fracture. Further treatment then depends on the degree of soft-tissue trauma as discussed in the section on open fractures.

Adult Fractures

Phalangeal Fractures:[12] Treatment of phalangeal fractures depends on the amount of displacement, and the phalanx involved. Distal phalanx fractures are usually of two types: 1) tuft fractures; and 2) avulsion of the dorsum at the insertion of the dorsal hood. The tuft fractures can usually be splinted without many problems. The avulsion fracture must be intraarticular, and treatment depends on the size of the avulsed fragment. A rule often followed is that if the fragment involves 30% or less of the articular surface of the DIPJ, then the fracture can be treated closed. If it involves more of the articular surface, and/or volar subluxation of the distal phalanx is also present, open treatment may be indicated to restore and maintain the articular congruity. In either case, immobilization can be accomplished with the DIPJ in slight extension to diminish tension on the extensor tendon.

Middle and proximal phalanx fractures can involve either the shaft, the base, or the head. Angulation and rotation may present problems. Angulation is caused by the pull of the flexor tendons and intrinsic muscles. Rotation may be difficult to recognize, but failure to correct abnormal rotation may allow the fracture to heal with a deformity of either overlapping or underlapping fingers. Rotation is evaluated by bending the fingers towards the palm and checking their position. Two points are usually checked: 1) the fingernails should lie in approximately the same plane; and 2) the fingers should point towards the scaphoid.

Most of these fractures can be treated closed by immobilizing the hand in the "position of safety," (Fig. 6-14) in which the MP joints are immobilized in 70-90 degrees flexion, and the PIPJ and DIPJ are flexed 10-20 degrees. This decreases tension on the intrinsics and, to a degree, the flexor tendons. Additionally, this position helps to prevent flexion contractures of the PIPJ and extension contractures of the MCPJ. Intraarticular fractures with large, single fragments many require open treatment to restore the articular surface.

Metacarpal Fractures (Non-Thumb):[12] Metacarpal fractures can occur through the head, the neck, the shaft, or the base of the metacarpal. Treatment varies according to the location of the fracture.

Metacarpal head fractures are often badly comminuted. In these cases, a short period of splinting followed by early, active motion, will hopefully mold the articular surface by using the soft tissue sleeve. The early motion will also help in preventing a stiff joint, but loss of motion is common after this difficult type of fracture.

Fractures through the neck and shaft of the metacarpals usually angulate with the apex dorsal. This is not a great problem in the fourth and fifth metacarpals because the corresponding CMC joints are quite mobile. However, the second and third CMC joints allow little motion, and any residual angulation of these bones will cause significant problems.

Most of these fractures are treated closed. The most common neck/shaft fractures occur in the fourth and fifth metacarpals (the so-called "boxer's fracture"), and opinion varies as to the amount of angulation which is acceptable. Some physicians accept up to 70 degrees of angulation, but 40 degrees is a more universally accepted figure. In the second and third metacarpals, because of the immobility of the adjacent CMC joints, angulation of over 10-15 degrees should be corrected.

Closed treatment of these fractures involves reducing them, usually by longitudinal traction and then using a method called the 90/90 technique. In this technique, the MCPJ and PIPJ are both flexed 90 degrees and the proximal phalanx is used to reduce the fracture by exerting a dorsally directed force on the distal fragment. Immobilization in this position, however, is not recommended, as the PIPJ will often develop a flexion contraction. Immobilization in the position of safety is usually adequate (Fig. 6-14).

Thumb Metacarpal:[12] Thumb metacarpal fractures can be treated closed if they are extraarticular. Because of the large amount of independent motion in the thumb, anatomic reduction is not necessary to achieve adequate motion, strength, and function. Although reduction should be attempted, if it cannot be maintained, some degree of angulation is acceptable.

Intraarticular fractures at the trapeziometacarpal joint are usually of two types. The most common fracture here is called a Bennett's fracture. In this fracture, the fracture line is oblique such that a triangular fragment at the ulnar base of the metacarpal remains attached to the trapezium with proximal displacement of the metacarpal. This fracture is unstable because of the pull of the abductor pollicis brevis (APB) on the base of the metacarpal, and the pull of the adductor pollicis (AdP) on the proximal phalanx. These two forces tend to lever the metacarpal away from the triangular fragment, by adducting and shortening the metacarpal. The current method of management favors percutaneous pinning of the fracture to maintain reduction, or possibly ORIF of the fracture.

The second type of trapeziometacarpal fracture is a Rolando's fracture. This is a comminuted intraarticular fracture at the base of the thumb metacarpal. The original description was for a T- or Y-shaped fracture pattern, but virtually all comminuted fractures in this location are now termed Rolando's fractures. Because of the comminution, these fractures are usually treated with a short period of immobilization, followed by early range of motion in an attempt to use the soft tissue sleeve to restore articular integrity. Occasionally, if the fracture is similar to the classic description, and the fragments are large enough, percutaneous pinning or ORIF may be preferred.

Scaphoid:[12,21] The scaphoid is the most commonly fractured carpal bone. The difficulty with the management of this fracture is the risk of nonunion and avascular necrosis. These complications are related to the peculiar blood supply of the scaphoid, which mainly enters the bone dorsolaterally and distally. Consequently, mid- or proximal scaphoid fractures will often be devascularized by the fracture.

In addition to an AP and lateral radiograph of the wrist, a scaphoid view is often obtained. This is an AP view of the wrist in ulnar deviation. Additional oblique views can also be ordered.

Nondisplaced fractures of the scaphoid are usually treated closed. The type of immobilization is controversial, however, and varies from a short-arm thumb spica excluding the thumb interphalangeal joint up to a long-arm thumb spica including the thumb IPJ and including the index and middle fingers. Because of this disparity, before deciding on a method of treatment, one should probably discuss this with either the senior resident or attending physician.

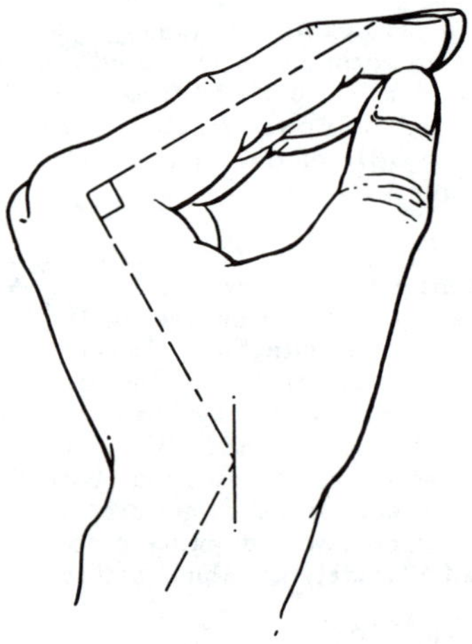

Fig. 6-14

"Safe" Position for Hand Splinting

Displaced fractures require reduction, which is not easily done without opening the fracture. A recent innovation in the treatment of scaphoid fractures has been the Herbert bone screw, which is a screw with two sets of threads of differing pitch and width, connected by a smooth shaft. Advancing the screw causes compression of the fracture site, because of the differing pitches of the screw. If closed reduction can be attained immobilization is adequate, but currently many orthopeadists favor the Herbert bone screw if the fracture site needs to be opened to achieve the reduction.

Distal Radius:[12,21,22] Fractures of the distal radius are quite common, the classic example being the Colles' fracture (see description above). Nondisplaced fractures are treated in a long-arm cast initially, often converted to a short-arm cast at 3-4 weeks.

The main problem with displaced fractures is shortening and angulation. In the normal lateral view of the distal radius, the articular surface has a volar tilt of about 10-13 degrees. In the typical Colles' fracture, the angulation causes the surface to tilt dorsally, and healing in this position will limit volar flexion at the wrist. In these cases, reduction should be attempted to restore the volar tilt, if possible. In older patients, with osteoporotic bone, the fracture is often comminuted and returning the distal radial surface to neutral is usually the best one can hope for. The radial length should be restored to diminish the deformity and allow maximum supination after fracture healing. Treatment after reduction is usually in a long-arm cast, excluding the thumb.

Younger patients with comminuted fractures will often have the fracture collapse with radial shortening in a cast. In these cases, an external fixator can be applied to maintain length while the fracture heals. Other options include percutaneous pin fixation or ORIF of the fracture, often applying a buttress-type plate to support the fracture.

Monteggia/Galeazzi:[21,22] A Monteggia fracture is a fracture of the ulnar shaft with a concomitant dislocation of the radial head. A Galeazzi fracture is a fracture of the radial shaft with a concomitant dislocation of the distal radio-ulnar joint. If there are no contraindications the recommended treatment in the adult for either fracture is closed reduction of the dislocation, with ORIF of the fracture. In a Galeazzi fracture, some physicians recommend maintaining the radioulnar reduction with a K-wire or pin.

It is imperative in forearm fractures that both the wrist and elbow be radiographed. Dislocation at one joint does not preclude concomitant dislocation at the other joint. Such a case would imply a complete disruption of the interosseous membrane and a severely unstable fracture.

Both-Bones Forearm:[22] Both-bone fractures of the forearm are, as the name implies, concurrent fractures of the shafts of the radius and ulna. In the adult, treatment is ORIF of both fractures, usually with plates and screws.

Olecranon:[21,22] Olecranon fractures will often be displaced because of the pull of the triceps on the proximal fragment. In those cases, the standard treatment is ORIF, using tension-band wire techniques. Nondisplaced fractures can occasionally be treated closed in a long-arm cast with the elbow in extension, or very slight flexion. This position cannot be maintained for more than a few weeks, however, because of the concern of loss of flexion at the elbow.

An alternative treatment in comminuted fractures of the olecranon is excision of the proximal fragment. Up to 80% of the olecranon can be excised without loss of elbow stability.

Radial Head:[19,22] Radial head fractures are classified as follows:

> Type I   -   Nondisplaced
> Type II -   Displaced, simple
> Type III -   Comminuted

Type I fractures are treated by a very short period of immobilization (long-arm cast or splint for 5-10 days) followed by early motion. Type III fractures are usually treated by excision of the radial head, if adequate reduction and internal fixation cannot be obtained.

The Type II fracture is controversial and each fracture requires individual assessment. A useful mnemonic to remember is the 3-3-3 rule: Openly reduce and internally fix the radial head if the articular surface is depressed 3 mm, if the fracture involves 30% of the articular surface, or if the fracture is angulated 30 degrees or more. Other options are replacement of the radial head with a prosthesis (currently controversial), or excision of the radial head, which is less desirable.

As a general rule, excision of the radial head is contraindicated if there is a concurrent wrist problem (chronic or acute), or if the elbow is unstable with damage to the medial collateral ligament of the elbow.

Distal Humerus (Intraarticular):[20,21,22] Distal humerus fractures are uncommon in the adult. Often the fracture will have a T- or Y-type configuration, with the longitudinal limb entering the joint. These are classified as follows:

> Type I   -   Nondisplaced
> Type II -   Displaced but not rotated
> Type III -   Displaced and rotated
> Type IV -   Severely comminuted

Type I fractures can be treated with immobilization in a long-arm cast for 3-4 weeks with early motion. In good operative candidates, the treatment of choice for Types II and III is ORIF. Type IV fractures often occur in the elderly and have the associated problem of osteoporotic bone. Treatment in the past has usually been by side-arm traction with an olecranon pin, a brief period of immobilization followed by early, active range of motion. Currently, ORIF is utilized in some cases if it appears that reduction and stabilization can be achieved.

Humeral Shaft:[22] Humeral shaft fractures can almost always be treated closed. Because of the mobility of the shoulder, if reduction cannot be maintained, a large degree of angulation (up to 20-25 degrees) can be accepted. In most cases the angulation will find the proximal fragment adducted by the pull of the pectoralis major. Reduction is then achieved by longitudinal traction and adduction of the distal fragment.

Immobilization can be of various types. Initial treatment in a coaptation splint is often adequate and keeps the patient comfortable for the first few days. After the swelling decreases, a prefabricated functional brace allows compression of the fracture by the soft-tissue envelope, maintaining the reduction and allowing elbow motion.

The main complication of this fracture is a radial nerve palsy. Therefore, the status of the radial nerve must always be evaluated and documented both before and after reduction of the fracture. A radial nerve palsy on presentation, i.e., as a consequence of the initial trauma, is **not** an indication to open the fracture and explore the nerve, as these virtually always resolve. If there are no clinical signs of radial nerve recovery, either by physical examination or by electrodiagnostic studies, within 2-4 months, surgical exploration of the radial nerve is indicated. Normal radial nerve function prior to reduction followed by loss of radial nerve function after reduction is, however, an indication to open the fracture site and explore the nerve.

Proximal Humerus:[7,22,24] Proximal humeral fractures have been classified by Neer as either nondisplaced, two-part, three-part or four-part fractures. The parts involved are the greater and lesser tuberosities, humeral shaft, and humeral head. The fracture between the shaft and head can occur either at the surgical or anatomic neck. To qualify as displaced the classification requires that a fragment be displaced one centimeter or angulated 45 degrees. Nondisplaced fractures can be treated with a shoulder immobilizer, followed by early motion when the pain subsides.

Two-part fractures include: 1) fracture at the surgical neck; 2) fracture at the anatomic neck; 3) avulsion of the greater tuberosity; and 4) avulsion of the lesser tuberosity, which is very rare as an isolated injury. Fracture at the surgical neck can usually be treated in a shoulder immobilizer, preceded by closed reduction, if needed. Early motion should be started once the patient is able to tolerate it. Fracture of the anatomic neck is quite rare by itself but is a difficult problem. Because the fracture is intraarticular, the risk of avascular necrosis of the humeral head is almost 90%. In the elderly, this fracture is probably an indication for insertion of a humeral head prosthesis. In younger patients, attempts should be made to save the head in hopes that necrosis will not occur. Since greater tuberosity fractures which are avulsed more than one centimeter will usually cause problems with subacromial impingement, this fracture should usually be treated with internal fixation.

Three-part fractures can include various combinations of any of the above four injuries. If significantly displaced, the age of the patient becomes critical.

In a young patient, if closed reduction is not possible, ORIF of the fracture is indicated. In the elderly, a humeral head hemiarthroplasty is usually the procedure of choice.

Four-part fractures usually occur in very osteoporotic bone and are uncommon except in the elderly. Recommended treatment is insertion of a humeral head prosthesis.

Clavicle:[22] Clavicle fractures can be classified according to their location - either medial third, middle third, or lateral third. Most of the these fractures should be treated by closed means. Even severely displaced fractures will usually heal, and the recommended treatment usually is a Figure-8 type harness to depress the medial fragment, which is usually elevated by the pull of the sternocleidomastoid muscle. Alternately, current studies are showing that treatment in a simple arm sling may give equivalent long-term results.

Upper Cervical Spine:[2] Fractures of the upper cervical vertebrae can be of several types. Recognition of fracture stability is of critical importance because of possible disastrous neurologic complications.

A <u>Jefferson fracture</u> is a fracture of the ring of C_1 (atlas), usually caused by an axial load to the top of the patient's head. These fractures do not impinge on the spinal canal and most patients are neurologically intact (if not, they are usually dead). Treatment is by halo collar and jacket for three months or until healing has occurred.

Fractures of the odontoid (dens) are classified as follows:

Type I - Avulsion fracture of the superior tip
Type II - Fracture through the isthmus of the odontoid
Type III - Fractures extending into the body of C_2

Types I fractures are stable and usually require no treatment. Type III fractures are unstable and usually are treated in a halo collar and jacket for three months. Type II fractures are also unstable. They are also often treated in a halo collar and jacket for three months. However, in Type II fractures, the rate of nonunion is significant (approximately 50%), and some physicians consider this an indication for open reduction and primary fusion of C_1 to C_2.

A <u>Hangman's fracture</u> is a fracture through the pedicles of C_2. The patient, if alive, is usually neurologically intact. The fracture is usually produced by an axial load to the head with the neck in an extended position. Treatment is immobilization in halo collar and jacket.

Lower Cervical Spine:[2,21] A common injury in the lower cervical spine is axial compression with the neck flexed, causing what is known as a teardrop fracture. Radiographically, the fracture has a small, triangular fragment at the antero-inferior margin of the vertebral body, similar in appearance to a teardrop. The name is also derived because the fracture is commonly associated with the devastating complication of immediate quadriplegia. Treatment is by halo collar and traction, if displaced, followed by immobilization in a halo jacket.

Flexion-rotation injuries to the cervical spine can cause dislocation of the vertebral bodies. In this injury, the facet joints dislocate, "jump" over one another, and become locked. Consequently, the injury is often described as jump-locked facets. The dislocation may be either unilateral or bilateral. If the dislocation is not complete, the facets may be said to be perched upon one another. Unfortunately, as one might expect, neurologic injuries are common with this injury. Unilateral jump-locked facets have a better prognosis, as the vertebral body cannot sublux forward more than 25% of the disk space, causing less cord impingement. Bilateral jump-locked facets usually cause at least 50% subluxation of the vertebral body.

Treatment of jump-locked or perched facets is reduction by halo traction and then placement of a halo jacket. The patient must be admitted to an intensive care unit or setting with one-to-one nursing care to monitor his neurologic status. Traction is applied using 10 lbs to counteract the weight of the head, and 5 lbs for each inter-space involved, starting with no more than 20 lbs <u>After placement of the weight, a lateral cervical radiograph and full neurologic exam is mandatory. If reduction does not occur, weight is then added in five-pound increments, in approximate half-hour intervals, being certain to repeat the lateral radiograph and the neurologic exam after each weight increase.</u> If reduction does not occur after using 35-40 lbs, open reduction and fusion is indicated .

Caution in handling and radiography of a patient with a suspected cervical spine injury is of critical importance. Handling of the patient is discussed in the chapter on Emergency Room techniques. A full radiographic evaluation of the cervical spine includes AP, lateral, obliques, and open-mouth odontoid views. **It is mandatory that the lateral view visualize the top of the T_1 vertebral body.** Otherwise, fractures or dislocations of lower vertebrae may be missed. Even if a more superior fracture is identified, there is a 10% incidence of a second fracture. Oblique radiographs are normally radiographed with the patient rolled to one side, which is not permissible until the spine is considered stable. An alternate technique is to keep the patient supine and have the radiologic technician angle the beam to obtain views which are termed "trauma obliques."

Ligamentous instability of the cervical spine can be as dangerous as osseous instability. White and Punjabi[2] have outlined criteria which allow radiographic estimation of ligamentous instability. When no fracture is identified, translation of the anterior border of two adjacent vertebral bodies by more than 4 mm on the lateral radiograph is indicative of significant ligamentous instability. On the lateral radiograph, angulation between the inferior borders of two adjacent vertebral bodies of more than 11 degrees is also consistent with ligamentous instability. However, because of the natural kyphos of the cervical spine, this angulation must be compared to neighboring interspaces for correct interpretation. An example is shown in Fig. 6-15. Treatment of ligamentous instability is controversial and should be discussed with the attending physician.

Often, no fracture or ligamentous injury can be seen on the radiographs, but cervical spine pain persists. In these cases, lateral flexion-extension views of

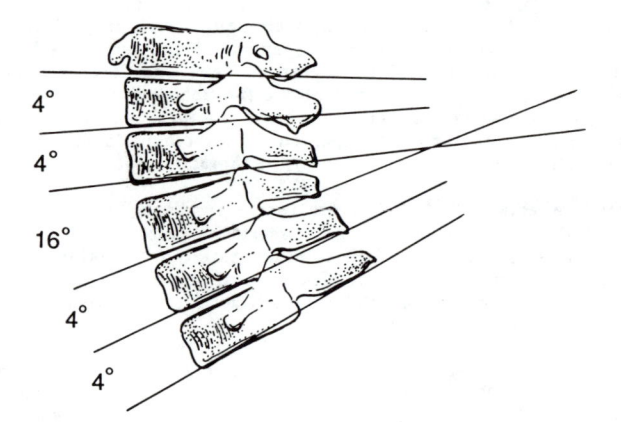

Fig. 6-15

The Method of Evaluating Ligamentous Instability of the Cervical Spine by Measuring the Angle Between the Lower Borders of Adjacent Cervical Vertebrae

the cervical spine can be obtained to evaluate stability. **Under no circumstances should the physician or any healthcare provider move the patient's neck for them.** The neck motion must be an active movement by the patient only. If there is too much pain to allow these views, presumptive evidence of soft-tissue injury exists and the patient should be placed in a semirigid collar until the pain has subsided enough to allow flexion-extension views.

Thoracolumbar Spine:[6,22] Thoracolumbar spine fractures are often discussed in terms of the three-column spine concept of Denis.[6] In this concept, the anterior one-half of the vertebral body constitutes the anterior column, the posterior one-half of the vertebral body constitutes the middle column, and the posterior elements (lamina, pedicles, processes) constitute the posterior column.

Compression fractures involve only the anterior column and are, as the name implies, noted by seeing compression of the anterior margin of the vertebral body. These are usually stable fractures and can be treated by bedrest and symptomatic treatment if there is no neurologic injury, which is rare. A common complication of these fractures is an ileus which should be watched for closely. These fractures are common in the elderly, with very osteoporotic bone. A compression fracture in a young, healthy person without significant trauma is highly suspicious of a pathologic fracture.

Burst fractures by definition involve the middle column. Radiographically, they are diagnosed by seeing either widening of the pedicles on the A-P radiograph, or posterior displacement of the posterior border of the vertebral body on the lateral radiograph. They are often associated with neurologic injury, are most common at the thoracolumbar border, and usually require surgical stabilization. Thoracic burst fractures are rare, but when they do occur, they are invariably accompanied by neurologic damage because of the relatively small size of the spinal canal in the thoracic spine.

Pelvic Fractures:[18,27] Pelvic fractures vary from the most innocuous of fractures to those possessing the highest mortality rates of any skeletal injury. Pelvic fractures are best classified as either stable or unstable. Features that make a pelvic fracture unstable are either disruption of the pubic symphysis by more than one inch, or disruption of the posterior sacroiliac ligaments, said to be the strongest ligaments in the body.

Unstable pelvic fractures possess high degrees of morbidity and mortality because the force necessary to create them also causes a significant amount of soft tissue damage. Pelvic hemorrhage associated with a pelvic fracture can be life-threatening. Exploration to control bleeding is indicated only as a last resort for two reasons: 1) it is extremely difficult, if not impossible to find and ligate a single source of bleeding; and 2) exploration often makes the situation worse by disrupting the tamponade caused by the expanding hematoma. In most cases, adequate control of bleeding can be achieved by application of an anterior external fixator which then compresses the two hemipelves, thereby decreasing the intrapelvic volume, and increasing the tamponade effect.

Further classification and treatment of pelvic fractures is a complex subject which cannot adequately be handled in this monograph. The interested reader is referred to either Tile's[27] or Mears' and Rubash's[18] books.

Acetabular Fractures:[18,27] Acetabular fractures, if displaced, carry a high risk of subsequent degenerative arthritis. The highest risk occurs in those fractures that involve the superior weightbearing surface of the acetabulum.

Acetabular fractures can be briefly classified as follows:

> Anterior wall fractures
> Anterior column fractures
> Posterior wall fractures
> Posterior column fractures
> Transverse fractures
> Complex fractures

The anterior and posterior wall of the acetabulum should be anatomically obvious. The anterior column is the bony strut running from the anterior superior iliac spine to the superior pubic ramus, and includes the anterior wall. The posterior column is the bony strut running from the posterior superior iliac spine to the inferior pubic ramus, and includes the posterior wall. Further classification and treatment is again a topic beyond the scope of this monograph.

Femoral Neck:[21,22] Femoral neck fractures cause a difficult problem because they are intraarticular and consequently carry a high risk of avascular necrosis of the femoral head. The most frequently used classification system is the Garden system, as follows:

Garden I	-	Impacted or incomplete fracture
Garden II	-	Complete, nondisplaced fracture
Garden III	-	Complete, partially displaced fracture
Garden IV	-	Complete fracture with total displacement

The risk of future avascular necrosis increases as the Garden grade increases.

Treatment of Garden I or II femoral neck fractures is usually by fixation in situ, using some type of threaded pins, placed inferior to the greater trochanter into the femoral neck and head.

Treatment of Garden III or IV femoral neck fractures depends, to a degree, on the age of the patient. In a relatively young patient, an attempt at reduction, followed by fixation in situ, may be indicated. In older patients, the treatment chosen is usually insertion of a femoral head prosthesis. In patients with preexisting acetabular disease, primary total hip arthroplasty is indicated.

Intertrochanteric:[21,22] Intertrochanteric fractures are the most common type of hip fractures and often occur in the very elderly. No universally accepted classification system exists. Treatment depends on the fracture pattern, degree of comminution, and medical condition of the patient.

Most intertrochanteric fractures are internally fixed by a sliding compression screw system. The compression screw enters the femur inferior to the greater trochanter and is threaded through a side plate, which is fixed to the proximal lateral femoral shaft. The compression screw works by its threads gaining purchase on the head and neck fragment, while being free to slide in the sleeve attached to the side-plate. This allows compression at the fracture site while maintaining relative stability. Complete stability of the fracture depends on the quality of the cortical bone on the medial (especially posteromedial) aspect of the proximal femur.

Subtrochanteric:[22] Subtrochanteric fractures are the rarest form of hip fracture and are often seen in pathologic conditions. They are defined as any fracture occurring between the lesser trochanter and a point five centimeters distal to it.

Several options for treatment exist, including fixation with a sliding compression screw with a long side plate, a blade plate which enters the femoral neck and attaches to a long side-plate, flexible intramedullary nails, and traction in the 90/90 degrees position. Another option is a rigid, crossed intramedullary nail device, the prototype of which is the Zickel nail.

Femoral Shaft:[21,22] Femoral shaft fractures can be treated in various manners. However, in the ideal situation, the treatment of choice is insertion of a rigid intramedullary nail. This often allows for immediate weightbearing and mobilization of the patient.

When the fracture is in the middle of the femoral shaft, or slightly proximal, the nail is often the only fixation needed. For very proximal, very distal, or comminuted fractures, special nails are made which accept screws both proximally and distally. These prevent rotation and shortening of the femur and are indicated in those situations.

Other methods of treatment of this fracture include placement of two long compression plates with screws, balanced skeletal traction, external fixation, and hip spica casts. These are less than optimal, and are chosen only when there is a relative contraindication to insertion of an IM nail, such as in Grade III open fractures, when there is neurovascular damage to the thigh, or when the patient's medical condition will not tolerate the operation.

Supracondylar Femur:[20,21,22] These fractures may or may not be intraarticular. Only the AO/ASIF classification system adequately describes these fractures but it is quite complex. The basic concern is the degree of comminution and the degree of displacement of articular surface of the distal femur.

Simple or mildly comminuted fractures with articular disruption are better treated with internal fixation. Several devices exist for this fracture, including a sliding compression screw device, blade plates with side plates, and a Zickel supracondylar device using flexible intramedullary rods.

If the fracture is too severely comminuted to allow fixation, other treatment options are skeletal traction and application of a cast brace with early motion.

Patella:[22] Simple patellar fractures are usually transverse. Treatment of these depends on the degree of displacement. Nondisplaced fractures can be treated in a long-leg cast with the knee in extension. Fractures displaced more than 2 mm or where there is a step-off of the articular surface more than 1 millimeter, should probably be treated by internal fixation. Current treatment favors fixation by tension band wiring.

Comminuted fractures may be treated either by a cast, excision of the fracture fragments, if small, or, in extreme cases, by patellectomy.

Tibial Plateau:[22] Tibial plateau fractures are classified as follows (Fig. 6-16):

Type I	-	Minimally displaced
Type II	-	Local compression
Type III	-	Split compression
Type IV	-	Total condylar depression
Type V	-	Bicondylar fracture

Treatment of these fractures is not specifically related to the classification. Instead, the key factor is the degree of irregularity of the articular surface of the knee. Depression of a portion of the articular surface of more then 5-8 millimeters is usually treated by open reduction with elevation of the fragments, bone grafting the defect, and some form of fixation - either screws, plates, or pins. Minimally displaced fractures are usually treated in a long-leg cast with weightbearing delayed until fracture healing is present radiographically.

Tibial Shaft:[17,20,22] The tibia is the most commonly fractured long bone in the body. Because the anteromedial surface of the tibia is almost subcutaneous, with minimal soft tissue covering, many tibial shaft fractures will be open, and these fractures cause a great deal of morbidity. The most important factors in predicting problems with healing of this fracture are the extent of soft-tissue damage, and the amount of initial fracture displacement.

Tibial shaft fractures can be treated with multiple methods, including skeletal traction (usually through the calcaneus), closed reduction/long-leg cast, pins and plaster, ORIF with plates and screws, ORIF with flexible intramedullary rods, ORIF with rigid intramedullary nails, and external fixation. Closed, rigid intramedullary nailing for unstable fractures is a current popular method treatment.

Most simple, stable, minimally displaced tibial shaft fractures can be treated by closed reduction, a long-leg cast, and non-weightbearing. Usually, this is worn for 6 weeks, and if there is evidence of healing, the cast is then changed to a patellar-tendon bearing (PTB) cast and full weightbearing is begun.

Predicting stability and judging the success of a closed reduction requires clinical experience. Basically, comminuted, segmental, spiral, and oblique fractures tend to be unstable with a tendency to shorten, angulate, and/or rotate. In relatively uncomplicated cases these probably still warrant an attempt at closed treatment. Frequent follow-up radiographs are needed, however, to be certain the reduction is maintained.

The closed reduction should satisfy several requirements. To fully evaluate the requirements it is important to obtain AP and lateral tib-fib radiographs which include both the knee and the ankle on the same radiograph cassette. The amount of bowing at the fracture site should then be measured on both the AP and lateral views. The tibia should: 1) have at least 50% cortical overlap at the fracture site; 2) be in < 10 degrees of varus/valgus when comparing the tibial plateau to the tibial plafond; and 3) have < 15 degrees of anterior or posterior bowing on the lateral film.

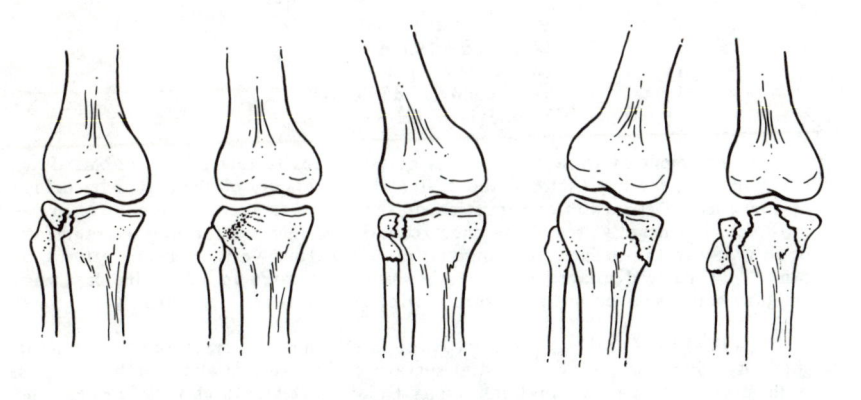

Fig. 6-16

Tibial Plateau Fractures

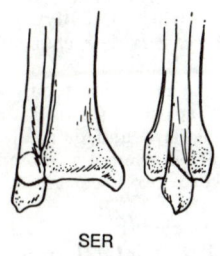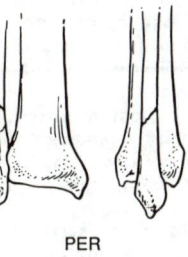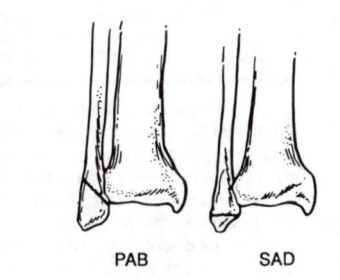

SER   PER   PAB   SAD

Fig. 6-17

Lauge-Hansen Classification

Any tibial shaft fracture for which these requirements cannot be met by closed treatment probably warrants internal or external fixation by one of the above methods. Further, any tibial fracture which on early follow-up radiographs proves unstable and fails these requirements should also be considered for open treatment or closed intramedullary nailing.

Ankle Fractures:[10,14,22] The classification of ankle fractures is quite complex. The most commonly used system is one devised by the Danish surgeon, Lauge-Hansen. Lauge-Hansen classifies ankle fractures into four (4) main types, as follows:

> Supination-External Rotation (SER)
> Supination-Adduction (SAD)
> Pronation-External Rotation (PER)
> Pronation-Abduction (PAB)

The first word above describes the position of the foot at the time of injury, while the second word(s) then describes the direction of the force causing the injury. Unfortunately, Lauge-Hansen then subdivided each of the above classifications, coming up with 13 categories of ankle fractures. This subclassification is probably not necessary to memorize, but to help in reduction of ankle fractures, it is important to be able to identify the above four main types. This identification can be done quite simply by studying the pattern of the fibular fracture (Fig. 6-17).

> SER - Spiral fibular fracture, distal end at the level of the tibial plafond
> PER - Spiral fibular fracture, distal end usually 4-7 cm above the tibial plafond
> SAD - Transverse fibular fracture at or below the level of the tibial plafond. If accompanied by a medial malleolar fracture, this will have an oblique pattern
> PAB - Oblique fibular fracture with distal end at the level of the tibial plafond. If accompanied by a medial malleolar fracture, this will have a transverse pattern

The Lauge-Hansen classification is used to aid in closed treatment of ankle fractures. The fracture can be reduced by reversing the mechanism of injury, which is described by the second word(s) in the classification system. Usually, the ankle is held in this position after reduction and placed in a long-leg cast in this position.

It is of equal importance, however, to evaluate the stability of an ankle fracture, and the Lauge-Hansen classification provides little help in this regard. For this situation it is more important to discuss a unimalleolar, bimalleolar, and trimalleolar classification. (Trimalleolar refers to the lateral and medial malleolus, as well as the posterior articular surface of the tibia, referred to as the posterior malleolus.)

Ankle stability is evaluated by examining the ankle mortise. The joint space between the talus and the tibial plafond should vary by no less than one millimeter on any side on the AP and mortise views of the ankle. A second method is to draw a line down the center of the tibia, and through the center of the talar dome on both the AP and lateral radiographs. These lines should be coincident or nearly so within 1 mm. If either parameter is not met, this implies that the talus has shifted in the mortise, and the fracture is potentially unstable. It also implies that it may be difficult to hold in a cast without internal fixation.

Most unimalleolar fractures will be stable. Only if the opposite malleolus has sustained severe ligamentous damage will the talus be able to shift. Most unimalleolar fractures can thus be handled in a closed manner.

Most bimalleolar fractures are unstable, as nothing is holding the talus in the mortise. An exception to this rule is when the fibular fracture is very low, below the level of the plafond, as it will block the talus and keep it centered in the mortise. Though these fractures may occasionally be held in a cast, more often they require ORIF.

Trimalleolar fractures imply severe soft tissue damage, a rotational injury, and are invariably unstable. Open reduction and internal fixation is indicated unless there is a specific contraindication.

Talus Fracture/Dislocations:[10,16,22] The talus can be fractured in several areas but the most common injury is to the talar neck. The Hawkins' classification system is used to describe these fractures:

Type I	-	Nondisplaced fracture of the talar neck without dislocation
Type II	-	Displaced fracture of the talar neck with subluxation or dislocation of the subtalar joint
Type III	-	Displaced fracture of the talar neck with dislocation of the body of the talus from both the subtalar and ankle joints

Because the blood supply to the talar dome enters through the talar neck, the main complication of this injury is avascular necrosis of the talar dome, with secondary degenerative arthitis of the tibiotalar joint. The risk of avascular necrosis increases with the severity of the injury. It is approximately 10% in Type I, 30% in Type II, and 90% in Type III injuries.

Type I fractures can be treated closed, usually in a short-leg cast with the foot in slight equinus. The leg is kept non-weightbearing for four weeks, and then weightbearing is allowed in the cast for another eight weeks or until healing is evident by radiograph.

Both Types II and III demand anatomic reduction of the talus. This is almost impossible to achieve by closed reduction and ORIF of these fractures is indicated.

Calcaneus Fractures:[16,22] Calcaneus fractures are usually caused by an axial load on the heel, often in a fall from a height. Because of the axial force transmission, a common accompanying injury (10%) is a compression fracture of the vertebral body. Many physicians will automatically obtain radiographs of the lumbosacral spine after this injury. At the least, the spine should be carefully examined to check for tenderness after this injury.

Calcaneus fractures are a difficult problem because of the common complication of degenerative arthritis of the subtalar joint. It would seem that the fracture would demand open reduction, but unfortunately the fracture is often so comminuted that it cannot be anatomically reduced even by open methods.

In addition to AP and lateral views of the foot, a special view of the calcaneus (Harris heel view) should be obtained. This is radiographed by angling the beam at 45 degrees from behind the leg, centering it on the posterior portion of the subtalar joint. To fully evaluate the extent of damage to the subtalar joint, the best imaging study is a CT scan. It is important to ask for coronal slices on the CT scan.

If the subtalar joint is shown not to be involved by the CT scan, or the fracture is deemed not reparable by open methods, it should be treated by non-weightbearing, initially in a long-leg cast.

Midfoot/Forefoot Fractures:[16,22] Multiple fracture types can occur in this region and several will be discussed. In the midfoot, the most common injury is what is called a Lisfranc fracture-dislocation. This is a rare fracture-dislocation through Lisfranc's joint, or the tarsometatarsal joint. Because the second metatarsal is the longest metatarsal proximally, it will often be fractured at its base, with the other metatarsals dislocated. Treatment of this fracture involves closed reduction and cross-pinning in situ, followed by application of a short-leg cast.

The base of the fifth metatarsal is frequently fractured and this injury tends to occur in two patterns. The first pattern, frequently seen in dancers, is an avulsion of the tip of the base caused by pull from the peroneus brevis muscle. It can be treated in a hard-sole cast shoe for comfort or, if the patient is in a great deal of pain, a short-leg cast or splint until the pain subsides.

The second pattern is a transverse fracture through the base of the fifth metatarsal, about 1-2 cm from the tip, known as a Jones' fracture. This fracture is usually treated in a short-leg cast. However, it has a high incidence of nonunion (50%), and primary internal fixation to avoid this complication may be preferred.

Although both patterns of fracture to the fifth metatarsal base are often called Jones' fractures, this eponym should be reserved for the second type described above. There is a definite difference in treatment and prognosis.

Fractures to the ends of the metatarsals and phalanges of the foot can usually be treated with a hard, wooden-soled cast shoe and allowing weight-bearing. For severely displaced metatarsal fractures, occasionally closed reduction and percutaneous pinning or ORIF with a plate and screws will be necessary to avoid a painful prominence on the plantar surface of the foot.

Adult Dislocations

Finger Dislocations:[12,22] Most finger dislocations can be recognized easily and reduced by the standard method of traction; exaggerate the mechanism, and reverse the mechanism. Radiographs should be obtained prior to reduction if there is any doubt that this is a fracture and not a dislocation.

Shoulder Dislocations:[7,22,24] Shoulder dislocations are common injuries in adolescents and young adults. The glenohumeral joint may dislocate anteriorly, posteriorly, inferiorly, and superiorly. By far the anterior glenohumeral dislocation is most common (95-98%). Posterior dislocations occur 2-4% of the time and the other dislocations are rarely seen.

Anterior glenohumeral dislocations usually occur when the arm is forcefully abducted and externally rotated. A common accompanying injury is to the axillary nerve; therefore sensation and motor function in this nerve should be documented both before and after reduction.

Multiple methods of closed reduction exist, but all use some method of traction on the arm in varying degrees of flexion and/or abduction. Reduction is almost impossible when the muscles are in severe spasm, and intravenous narcotics and muscle relaxants are usually needed to allow the person to relax enough to allow reduction. After reduction, the arm should be placed in a shoulder immobilizer with the forearm across the chest. The length of immobilization is very controversial, varying from 1-2 days (until pain subsides) up to six weeks.

Anterior glenohumeral dislocations frequently become recurrent. This is especially so in the adolescent age group, where the incidence of recurrence is as high as 90%. Once the dislocation occurs a second time in this age group, the chance of frequent recurrence is almost 100%. Therefore, in adolescents, a second dislocation is usually an indication for open reconstruction of the shoulder to prevent further recurrences.

Posterior glenohumeral dislocations are rarely seen, but are commonly missed (50-75%). This is often due to a failure to obtain a complete x-ray series of the shoulder. The two important views to document posterior dislocation, if suspected, are an axillary lateral and a Y-scapular lateral. Without these views, this injury will often not be diagnosed, leading to considerable morbidity.

The posterior dislocation occurs by a mechanism of forceful adduction and internal rotation (a common position in a seizure). The diagnosis should be suspected whenever a patient has injured his shoulder and cannot externally rotate his hand to the neutral position. In addition a mass will often be palpable posteriorly.

Acromioclavicular Dislocations:[7,22] An acromioclavicular (A-C) dislocation is colloquially known as a shoulder separation. It is usually caused by a blow to the top of the shoulder, and is often seen in contact sports.

The scapula is fixed to the clavicle by two sets of ligaments: 1) the acromioclavicular ligaments; and 2) the coracoclavicular ligaments. A-C dislocations are graded by the amount of damage to these ligaments.

Type I A-C dislocations imply a sprain of the joint without a complete tear of either ligament. A Type II injury implies a tear of the acromioclavicular ligaments with the coracoclavicular ligaments intact. Because the coracoclavicular ligaments provide stability in the coronal plane, this injury will not show marked elevation of the lateral end of the clavicle. However, that is the pattern seen in a Type III injury where both sets of ligaments are torn.

If there is a question about the degree of an A-C dislocation, stress radiographs can be obtained. These are filmed with 10-15 lbs suspended from both wrists by a strap (not held in the hands). Both A-C joints must be seen on the same film. Elevation of one joint by 5 mm or more implies a severe Type II or Type III dislocation.

Treatment of the Type I injury is symptomatic. The patient should be given a sling for comfort for a few days but can usually begin exercising his shoulder in 1-2 days and should be encouraged to do so. Treatment of the Type II and III injuries is more controversial. Some physicians recommend internal fixation of Type III injuries and a few will recommend repair of both types of injuries. More commonly, these are treated with special harnesses which pull down the lateral end of the clavicle to keep the A-C joint reduced.

Elbow Dislocations:[19,22] Most elbow dislocations occur from a fall on an outstretched hand. By far the most common pattern is a posterior dislocation, where the coronoid process is dislocated posterior to the distal humerus. Reduction is usually easily performed by gentle longitudinal traction and flexion. The deformity should not be grossly exaggerated as this can place stress on the neurovascular structures anterior to the elbow. A posterior splint and sling should be used for 1-2 weeks but active motion should then be encouraged to prevent an elbow flexion contracture from developing. Recurrent instability is very uncommon.

Hip Dislocations:[22] Hip dislocations usually result from major trauma. Sciatic and femoral nerve damage can occur, and neurologic exam should be carefully documented. Because of concern about continued pressure on the neurovascular structures, reduction should be obtained as quickly as possible. A common mechanism of this injury is an automobile accident where the passenger's flexed knee strikes the dashboard, driving the femoral head posteriorally and often fracturing the posterior acetabular wall.

Posterior dislocation is the most common type, occurring in about 85% of the cases. Because of the large muscles about the hip, and the pain and spasm involved, general anaesthesia is usually required for reduction. Reduction is achieved by adduction, flexion and traction, followed by abduction and external rotation. A common complication of this injury is avascular necrosis of the femoral head which occurs in about 10% of the cases and may occur as late as three years after the injury.

Anterior dislocations are fairly rare. Again, general anaesthesia is often required for reduction, which can be achieved by traction, extension and internal rotation of the hip.

A special problem is dislocation of total hip prostheses. The direction of dislocation will vary in these cases according to the surgical approach used. As in dislocations of the native femoral head, these can cause neurologic problems and reduction should be achieved quickly, if possible. If the dislocation is more than 1-2 days old, this will often require skeletal traction on the limb to decrease the contracture of the abductor musculature. After reduction, the patient is usually placed in a hip spica cast with the lower extremity flexed and abducted slightly. Recurrent dislocations of a total hip prosthesis may be an indication to revise the prosthesis.

Knee Dislocations: Knee dislocations are an orthopaedic emergency because of the high incidence of vascular damage to the limb. The dislocation is usually obvious if the physician has seen one previously. In those cases, the knee should be reduced immediately, even before proceeding to radiology, to reduce pressure on the vascular supply to the lower leg. If pedal pulses are absent after reduction, immediate exploration of the popliteal artery is indicated. If the surgeon elects to obtain an arteriogram, this should be done in the operating room. This is because, after a knee dislocation, delay of more than six hours in restoring the vasculature is associated with a very high incidence of above-knee amputations.

If the pedal pulses are intact, an arteriogram of the lower extremity should still be obtained to be certain that vascular reconstructive surgery is not needed. If the arteriogram is normal, the leg should be placed in a long-leg splint, but it must be watched carefully for a developing compartment syndrome. In addition, vascular insufficiency to the leg can still occur via late arterial thrombosis, and the vascular supply to the leg should be checked carefully.

Ligament reconstruction to the severely damaged knee may be performed acutely but is often performed on a delayed basis.

Pediatric Fractures

Pediatric Both-Bones Forearm:[21,23] Unlike in the adult situation, both-bones fractures in children can be treated successfully closed. Reduction is usually achieved by placing a hematoma block into both bones, and reducing each bone individually. The arm should be placed in a long-arm cast or splint.

The rotational position of the wrist in the cast varies with the position of the fracture. Most proximal third fractures will need to be immobilized in slight pronation, most middle third fractures should be placed in neutral, and most distal third fractures will require immobilization in slight supination. However, postreduction films to evaluate the rotational position of the arm should be obtained, and the reduction adjusted accordingly.

Pediatric Condylar Elbow:[23] Condylar fractures of the elbow in children, most commonly of the lateral condyle, are usually caused by a fall on the outstretched arm. The fracture is intraarticular and, if significantly displaced (>2 millimeters), should be treated by open reduction and fixation with smooth pins. Nondisplaced fractures can be treated by immobilization in a long-arm cast, but frequent radiographs are needed to be certain displacement does not occur.

Pediatric Supracondylar Elbow[21,23] This is a very common fracture in the pediatric population and one of the most difficult fractures to treat. Most of these fractures occur from a fall on an outstretched arm. Neurovascular injuries are common, and ischemic contractures of the forearm muscles can occur if the injury is treated incorrectly. Most of these fractures have the distal fragment displaced posteriorly, known as an extension-type injury.

Nondisplaced fractures can be treated initially by immobilization in a long-arm splint with the elbow flexed. Flexion of up to 120 degrees renders the fracture more stable but also increases the risk of neurovascular compromise. In nondisplaced fractures the elbow should probably be flexed no more than 90 degrees.

Minimally displaced fractures can be reduced by flexing the arm, usually to greater than 90 degrees. After application of a splint the neurovascular status of the arm and postreduction radiographs must be evaluated. **If neurovascular compromise has occurred, the arm must be flexed less, extending the elbow until the neurovascular status of the limb returns to normal. <u>Postreduction radiographs should again be checked, and if the reduction is lost in this position, this is an absolute indication for open reduction and pinning, or closed reduction and percutaneous pinning under adequate anaesthesia. The important point is to maintain stability of the fracture while the elbow is extended enough to preserve the neurovascular function of the upper extremity</u>.**

Grossly displaced fractures usually require open reduction and pinning of the fracture or percutaneous pinning of the fracture under fluoroscopic guidance. An alternative treatment is Dunlap's-type traction or overhead traction to achieve reduction followed by a long-arm cast.

Because of the danger of the disastrous complication of neurovascular injury to the limb, with the sequelae of a forearm muscle necrosis, most patients with this injury, if it is displaced at all, should be admitted to the hospital for 24-48 hours for observation.

The most common complication after this injury is development of a cubitus varus deformity ("gunstock deformity") at the elbow. It is essentially a cosmetic deformity which is usually not of functional significance. It is important, however, to advise and reassure the parents early about this possible problem.

Proximal Humeral Physeal Injuries:[7,23] Eighty percent of the longitudinal growth of the humerus occurs in the proximal humeral physis. Consequently, an injury to this physis is of great clinical significance. However, this large percentage of growth allows tremendous remodelling of the proximal humerus if not reduced perfectly.

Most of these injuries are either Salter I or II fractures. Operative treatment is rarely indicated. In children with displaced fractures, reduction should be attempted by traction and gentle manipulation. In very young children, if reduction is successful, it can usually be maintained with a shoulder immobilizer. After the age of five, displaced fractures will tend to redisplace if the arm is placed in a shoulder immobilizer. Reduction and treatment in this age group is often achieved via overhead traction in the "salute position" (the arm is placed in the position one makes when saluting). After reduction, if the fracture is unstable when moved from the salute position, a shoulder spica cast must be placed with the arm remaining in the salute position.

Pediatric Hip Fractures:[21,23] Pediatric hip fractures usually occur from major trauma and are a difficult problem. They are classified as follows:

Transphyseal fractures
Femoral neck (cervical) fractures
Cervicotrochanteric fractures
Intertrochanteric fractures

Injury to the proximal femoral physis carries the ominous prognosis of 100% certainty of developing avascular necrosis of the femoral head. If displaced at all, the treatment is prompt reduction with internal fixation with threaded pins through the femoral neck.

Current thinking on the other three types of injury also favors open fixation with threaded pins followed by placement of a hip spica cast until healing occurs. Intertrochanteric fractures can be treated simply by the cast or by traction followed by the spica cast, but internal fixation allows earlier mobilization.

The two main complications of these fractures are: 1) avascular necrosis of the femoral head with development of degenerative arthritis; and 2) coxa vara. Internal fixation has not been shown to decrease the incidence of avascular necrosis, but definitely decreases the risk of developing coxa vara.

Pediatric Femoral Shaft:[21,23] Treatment of pediatric femoral shaft fractures has changed in the past few years. It was previously recommended that the injury be treated with traction followed by application of a spica cast. In the older pediatric age groups (> 5 yrs), this still may be necessary to achieve an adequate reduction of the fracture. However, in the very young, even severely displaced femoral shaft fractures will remodel, and immobilization in a hip spica cast is all that is necessary. Current treatment includes external fixation in selected patients.

Distal Femoral Physeal Injuries:[21,23] Injury to the distal femoral physis can cause a number of complications. The most common mechanism is hyperextension causing the epiphysis to be displaced anteriorly. With this injury, the neurovascular structures are at risk and need to be carefully evaluated. Most of these fractures will be Salter I or Salter II types.

Treatment for the Salter I or Salter II injury is closed reduction and application of a long-leg cast with the knee flexed. The amount of flexion is determined by placing the knee in the "safe zone" between too much flexion, risking vascular compression, and too little flexion, risking redisplacement. Open reduction is seldom indicated; however, percutaneous pinning with Steinman pins for stabilization is a recommended procedure, as redisplacement can occur, even in a long-leg cast.

A common complication of this injury is growth plate arrest. Although usually not common after Salter I or Salter II injuries, there is a 50% incidence of this complication in fractures of the distal femoral physis. Consequently, the parents need to be warned that this complication is a possibility. In addition, the child should be examined yearly until skeletal maturity is reached.

Other Musculoskeletal Injuries

Almost all acute soft-tissue injuries can be treated by remembering the mnemonic *PRICE*:

P	-	Protection
R	-	Rest
I	-	Immobilization
C	-	Compression
E	-	Elevation

All of these are important to prevent further injury to the area, and to decrease the swelling which lengthens the rehabilitation period.

Wrist Injuries:[12] The causes of soft-tissue pain at the wrist are myriad, and include ligamentous injuries, cartilage tears, tendinitis, arthritis, and nerve inflammation. Each will be briefly discussed.

Ligament injuries usually involve the volar radiocarpal ligaments and can cause chronic wrist pain. Diagnosis is made by tenderness over the volar wrist capsule, supported by clinical and radiographic evidence of carpal instability. This is a complex topic and must be considered, as it often requires a special series of radiographs, arthrography, or arthroscopy to demonstrate the problem. Treatment in chronic cases is controversial but may begin with splinting and nonsteroidals. If this fails, ligament reconstruction has inconsistent results, and various wrist arthrodeses or resection arthroplasties may be selected. Effective treatment of ligament damage requires diagnosis at the time of injury. This again necessitates a high degree of suspicion so that the proper radiographs may be obtained.

Cartilage tears within the wrist capsule usually involve the triangular fibrocartilage complex, a meniscal-like structure in the ulnar side of the wrist capsule. In addition to pain in the area, rotation of the wrist joint will often produce a palpable or audible click. The diagnosis can be confirmed by arthrography or arthroscopy of the wrist. During arthroscopy, the torn portion of the triangular fibrocartilage can be resected, and this will often effect a cure.

Tendinitis can involve many of the tendons about the wrist, but most commonly the tendons in the anatomic snuffbox will become inflamed, causing a condition known as DeQuervain's tenosynovitis. Diagnosis is made by tenderness over the extensor tendons of the first dorsal compartment (AbPL and EPB), inflammation noted in that area (they are very superficial), and a positive Finkelstein's test. Finkelstein's test is performed by asking the patient to make a fist over his thumb, and ulnarly deviating the wrist. Often the thumb-in-fist is itself acutely painful in this condition and the patient will not ulnarly deviate the wrist.

DeQuervain's tenosynovitis must be differentiated, especially in older age groups, from degenerative arthritis at the trapeziometacarpal joint. The test to differentiate the two is the grind test, which will usually be negative in DeQuervain's but positive in degenerative arthritis. It is performed by holding the thumb proximal phalanx and MCPJ in the examiner's hands and forcefully pushing against the trapeziometacarpal joint, while also rotating it slightly, to cause a grinding motion.

Treatment of DeQuervain's and trapeziometacarpal arthritis both begin with nonsteroidal anti-inflammatants and immobilizing the thumb in a thumb spica splint. Both may also respond to local injections with corticosteroids. Advanced chronic arthritis of the trapeziometacarpal occasionally will require a fusion, trapezial prosthesis, or by resection of the trapezium and replacement with a rolled tendon ("anchovie procedure").

The most common compression neuropathy at the wrist is carpal tunnel syndrome. This is a compression of the median nerve at the wrist by the transverse carpal ligament. The most common cause is flexor tenosynovitis in the carpal tunnel. The diagnosis is made by symptoms of pain at the wrist or hand, numbness or paraesthesias in the median nerve distribution, a positive Phalen's or Tinel's test. The diagnosis can be confirmed by nerve conduction studies. Phalen's test consists of holding the wrist in volar flexion for up to a minute. Often this will reproduce the paraesthesias in the radial three and one-half digits. Tinel's test is performed by gentle tapping over the median nerve at the wrist; a positive test will also elicit the appropriate paraesthesias in the median nerve distribution of the hand.

Treatment of carpal tunnel syndrome begins with nonsteroidal medication and wrist splinting. Later treatment can include injecting the carpal tunnel with a steroid preparation, but this should not be repeated for fear of tendon rupture. Resistant cases can be treated surgically by dividing the transverse carpal ligament to decompress the median nerve.

Gamekeeper's Thumb:[12] Gamekeeper's thumb is an injury to the ulnar collateral ligament of the thumb MCP joint, causing instability at that joint. It was formerly seen in British gamekeepers who stretched out the ligament by wringing off the heads of rabbits, but today it is most commonly seen in skiiers and basketball players.

The stability of the MCP joint should be tested by applying an ulnarly directed force to the joint, both with the joint extended and flexed. The joint should be tighter in flexion than extension. Comparison to the opposite thumb is necessary because people have such varying joint stability and ligamentous laxity. A joint that opens up less than 35 degrees when compared to the opposite thumb has probably not suffered a complete rupture of the ligament. In this case, treatment would be a short-arm cast with a thumb spica.

A joint that, under stress, deviates 35 degrees ulnarly more than the opposite thumb, especially in flexion, probably implies a complete rupture of the ulnar collateral ligament. Most hand surgeons recommend open repair of the ligaments in those cases, because of the failure to heal from closed treatment.

The main complication is failure of the ligament to heal and resulting instability of the joint. In a complete rupture, this will often be caused by interposition of the adductor pollicis tendon between the two ends of the ligament, known as a Stener's lesion. The incidence of this lesion varies in different reports but is of high enough frequency that it leads many physicians to operate when they believe a complete rupture of the ligament exists.

Impingement Syndromes/Rotator Cuff Tears:[7,24] Impingement syndrome is the term used to describe pain in the subacromial space when the humerus is elevated or internally rotated. This causes compression of the rotator cuff and subacromial bursa against the undersurface of the acromion and coracoacromial ligament. The elevation is classically forward flexion but abduction will often cause a similar pain. The pain will often become worse at night, as the subacromial bursa becomes hyperemic after a day of activity. Diagnosis is confirmed by the <u>impingement sign</u> (pain which occurs after forward flexing the arm to 90 degrees, and forcefully internally rotating the shoulder) and the impingement test. The <u>impingement test</u> is performed by first eliciting a positive impingement sign. Five milliliters of Xylocaine are then injected into the subacromial space, and the impingement sign is again sought. Relief of pain after injection confirms that the subacromial space was indeed the source of pain.

Impingement syndrome is an overuse syndrome which is often exacerbated by certain anatomic variations in the acromion. Treatment consists of activity modification, avoiding those activities which are done overhead, if possible. In early cases, nonsteroidal medication will often relieve the inflammation and effect a cure.

Chronic cases are often treated by injection of a preparation consisting of a steroid and a long-acting local anaesthetic. It is important to inject only into the subacromial space and not the tendons of the rotator cuff, because of the risk of tendon rupture. Injection is performed under completely sterile conditions at all times. The lateral surface of the acromion is palpated and the needle inserted through the skin until it strikes the acromion. The needle is "walked-down" the acromion until the needle passes under the acromion - it will then be in the subacromial space - and the solution is then injected.

The subacromial space should not be injected with steroids more than twice, because of the risk of tendon rupture. Cases that do not respond to the above conservative measures after six months of treatment are candidates for surgery. The procedure of choice is an anteroinferior acromioplasty combined with division of the coracoacromial ligament.

Chronic rotator cuff tears are the end stage of impingement syndrome, in which the continued pressure over the tendons passing through the subacromial space, finally causes them to rupture. Differentiation from pure impingement syndrome is difficult clinically, but one test that can be used is the drop-arm test. With the affected arm elevated 90 degrees in the plane of the scapula, and internally rotated fully, pressure on the arm will cause it to drop dramatically. Theoretically, this position isolates the supraspinatus, the most commonly ruptured tendon of the cuff. However, a strong deltoid muscle can overcome this resistance and the test is neither sensitive nor specific.

Accurate diagnosis of a rotator cuff tear demands either an arthrogram or, in the proper hands, an ultrasonographic examination of the shoulder. If a tear is documented, therapy must be individualized to the patient and his lifestyle. Often, tears will become asymptomatic with conservative therapy, and a short course is appropriate. If a patient has been compliant with conservative therapy for six months, remains symptomatic, and has a documented rotator cuff tear, surgical repair of the cuff should be offered to the patient as an option.

Tennis Elbow:[19] "Tennis elbow" is the term popularly used to describe tendinitis about the origin of the extensor muscles from the lateral epicondyle of the humerus. The term originated because it is often seen in tennis players, but it is an overuse syndrome that can be caused by many other activities.

Treatment is initially directed at decreasing the frequency of the activity causing the problem, often tennis. After the acute event resolves, the patient may resume the activity, but should be advised to alter the biomechanics of the activity to take stress off the elbow. For tennis players, this often involves lessons to improve the mechanics of the patient's/player's strokes.

Nonsteroidal medication will also decrease the inflammation in the area, as will ice packs to the elbow after performing the exacerbating activity. A forearm brace that compresses the extensor musculature just distal to the elbow often provides dramatic relief in difficult cases. This works by transferring the effective origin of the extensor muscles to just below the brace, rather than from the lateral epicondyle. Surgery is reserved for only the most recalcitrant cases. Corticosteroid injections are controversial, as they frequently provide relief, but may put the muscle origins at risk for degeneration and possible rupture.

Low Back Strain:[26] This is a universally common malady and one which is sometimes difficult to manage. Low back pain causes more missed work days than any other medical problem and nationally is a significant economic problem. It is important to be certain that one is dealing "only" with a soft tissue strain, by thorough assessment to rule out herniated disc, fractures, spinal tumors, abdominal aortic aneurysms, renal problems, gynecologic problems, and low back pain associated with new onset, or progressive, neurologic dysfunction (to name a few other sources of low back pain).

In the past, treatment of an acute low back strain has included strict bedrest for 1-2 weeks, treatment with nonsteroidal anti-inflammatory medication and muscle relaxants, and application of hot packs to the back. Recent studies have shown no difference in eventual function between early mobilization and strict bedrest for two weeks.[8,11] In addition, the use of muscle relaxants is no longer felt to be indicated.

Current therapy emphasizes patient education which is important in acute low back injuries to avoid the development of a chronic problem. In the acute situation, a few days (not more than 3-4) of bedrest, followed by gradual resumption of daily activities is currently recommended. In addition, non-steroidal medication and hot packs continue to be helpful in most patients.

For long-term protection, the patient should be advised that a program of alternating rest and exercise is important - both to rest the inflamed muscles in the area, and to keep the muscles in proper tone. The patient should also be taught the importance of proper posture, weight control, and lifestyle alterations in lifting and moving. Weight control is especially important, as it reduces stress on the lumbosacral spine.

Knee Injuries:[10,21,22] Many times a patient will incur what appears to be a significant knee injury, but no fracture or dislocation will be seen. It is important in these cases to document the presence of a knee effusion and the chronologic development of the effusion.

Without a fracture, most (85%) significant acute knee effusions are indicative of acute rupture of the anterior cruciate ligament. If this has occurred, the effusion will develop quickly, within the first few hours, because of the vascularity of the anterior cruciate. Another, less common, cause of a knee effusion is rupture of the patellar retinaculum, so the integrity of the quadriceps mechanism must be examined carefully.

Effusions that develop more slowly (over 24 hours) are usually indicative of a less severe injury, often seen in meniscal or osteochondral injuries.

Effusions from meniscal injuries will often not be significantly bloody, and if in doubt, aspiration of the joint can be undertaken.

Swelling about the knee does not necessarily indicate an effusion. Localized swelling with local tenderness will be seen with isolated injuries to the collateral ligaments.

Documentation of an acute knee effusion is quite important because it usually implies anterior cruciate ligament damage. Attempting to examine the knee for anterior instability is often impossible in the acute situation, because of the degree of pain and spasm. Aspiration of the effusion, with injection of local anaesthetic will often allow a better exam and provide more comfort to the patient. This should be followed by placing the injured leg in a knee immobilizer. Weightbearing is permissible, although the patient may not tolerate this well, so crutches should be prescribed.

If the knee definitely shows instability consistent with anterior cruciate damage, surgical reconstruction should be considered in young, active individuals. The patient should be evaluated promptly by an orthopaedist familiar with cruciate ligament reconstruction, as this reconstruction is more successful if done before secondary instabilities develop.

If the exam is equivocal, the patient should periodically be evaluated by an orthopaedist, as follow-up exams may document instability as the pain and muscle spasm subside.

Knees with collateral ligament injuries and meniscal injuries may also be treated initially with placement in a knee immobilizer. After the initial pain from the injury subsides, the patient should be taught quadriceps and hamstring strengthening exercises to help rehabilitate the knee. If these are isolated injuries, this may be all that is needed. However, these patients should be followed-up closely because both injuries can cause long-term disabilities.

Ankle Sprains:[14,21] Ankle sprains are most commonly caused by inversion injuries to the ankle; hence, the ligament damage is usually on the lateral side of the ankle.

Three ligaments support the lateral side of the ankle: 1) the anterior talofibular ligament; 2) the calcaneofibular ligament; and 3) the posterior talofibular ligament. They are most often injured in that order.

Swelling about the lateral malleolus with tenderness about the anterior talofibular ligament indicates at least a Grade I ankle sprain, implying slight stretching of the ligament without disruption. Grade II ankle sprains imply partial tearing of a ligament, while a Grade III sprain is consistent with complete rupture of a ligament, usually the anterior talofibular ligament.

Ankle stability can be evaluated by performing an ankle drawer test. To perform this test, place one hand around the heel, with the thumb on the talus. The other hand is placed just above the ankle joint to stabilize the tibia. While the tibia is stabilized, place the foot in slight plantar flexion and internal rotation, and then pull forward with the hand behind the heel. Stability can be strictly determined only by comparing the injured ankle to the contralateral ankle. Because the calcaneofibular and posterior talofibular ligaments are rarely ruptured, significant ankle instability is rare from an acute injury and can occur only in a Grade III injury. If present, it is best treated in a short-leg cast. Ligament reconstruction in chronic cases of ankle instability may be indicated.

Grade II and Grade III ankle sprains will often be quite painful. In those cases the patient will usually be more comfortable if treated for several days in a posterior splint, followed by resumption of full weightbearing. Grade I injuries can be treated with weightbearing as tolerated and nonsteroidal anti-inflammatory medication.

References

1. Carter DR. "Biomechanics of bone fracture." in *Orthopaedic Surgery Update Series*, Vol. 1, No. 1, 1982.
2. Cervical Spine Research Society. *The Cervical Spine*. Philadelphia: J. B. Lippincott, 1983.
3. Charnley JS. *The Closed Treatment of Common Fractures*. Edinburgh: E & S Livingston, 1968.
4. Crenshaw AH, ed. *Campbell's Operative Orthopaedics*. 7th Edition. 4 vols. St. Louis: C. V. Mosby, 1987.
5. Dahlin DC, Unni KK. *Bone Tumors*. 4th edition. Champaign: C. C. Thomas, 1986.
6. Denis F. The three column spine and its significance in the classification of acute thoracolumbar spinal injuries. *Spine*, 8(8): 817-831, 1983.
7. DePalma AF, ed. *Surgery of the Shoulder*. 3rd edition. Philadelphia: J. B. Lippincott, 1983.
8. Deyo RA, Diehl AK, Rosenthal M. How many days of bed rest for acute low back pain? A randomized clinical trial. *N Engl. J. Med.*, 315: 1064-1070, 1986.
9. Enneking WF. *Musculoskeletal Tumor Surgery*. 2 vols. New York: Churchill-Livingstone, 1983.
10. Evarts CMcC, ed. *Surgery of the Musculoskeletal System*. 4 vols. Philadelphia: Churchill-Livingstone, 1985.
11. Frymoyer JW. Back pain and sciatica, *N Engl. J. Med.*, 318: 291-300, 1988.
12. Green DP, ed. *Operative Hand Surgery*. 2nd edition. 3 vols. New York: Churchill-Livingstone, 1987.
13. Huvos AG. *Bone Tumors: Diagnosis, Treatment and Prognosis*. Philadelphia: W. B. Saunders, 1979.
14. Kelikian H, Kelikian AS. *Disorders of the Ankle*. Philadelphia: W. B. Saunders, 1985.
15. Madewell JE, et al. Radiologic and Pathologic Analysis of Solitary Bone Lesions: Part I: Internal Margins, pp. 715-748; Part II: Periosteal Reactions, pp. 749-784; Part III: Matrix Patterns, pp. 750-785., in *Radiologic Clinics of North America*, December 1981, Vol. 19, Number 4.

16.   Mann RA, ed. *Surgery of the Foot*. 5th edition. St. Louis: C. V. Mosby, 1986.
17.   Mears DC. *External Skeletal Fixation*. Baltimore: Williams & Wilkins, 1983.
18.   Mears DC, Rubash HE. *Pelvic and Acetabular Fractures*. Thorofare, NJ: Slack, 1986.
19.   Morrey BF, ed. *The Elbow and Its Disorders*. Philadelphia: W. B. Saunders, 1985.
20.   Mueller ME, Allgoewer M, Schneider R, Willenegger H. *Manual of Internal Fixation*. Berlin: Springer-Verlag, 1979.
21.   Orthopaedic Knowledge Update 2. Home Study Syllabus. Chicago: American Academy of Orthopaedic Surgeons, 1987.
22.   Rockwood CA, Green DP, eds. *Fractures In Adults* . 2nd edition. 2 vols. Philadelphia: J. B. Lippincott, 1984.
23.   Rockwood CA, Wilkins KE, King RE, eds. *Fractures In Children*. Philadelphia: J. B. Lippincott, 1984.
24.   Rowe CR, ed. *The Shoulder*. New York: Churchill-Livingstone, 1988.
25.   Schajowicz F. *Tumors and Tumorlike Lesions of Bone and Joints*. New York: Springer-Verlag, 1981.
26.   Spengler DM. *Low Back Pain: Assessment and Management*. New York: Grune & Stratton, 1987.
27.   Tile M. *Fractures of the Pelvis and Acetabulum*. Baltimore: Williams & Wilkins, 1984.

Chapter 7

Casting and Splinting Techniques

The goal of casting and splinting is to immobilize the injured extremity for comfort and maintain adequate alignment of fractures and/or ligamentous structures for healing to occur. Satisfactory immobilization and alignment may initially be obtained with splinting although splints tend to loosen with time and require more frequent adjustments.

Casting and splinting materials[2]: The time-honored casting material is plaster of Paris. The plaster of Paris bandage consists of a roll of fabric (originally crinoline, now a fabric called leno) which is impregnated with plaster of Paris. The addition of water to calcium sulfate causes it to be transformed into its crystalline form (gypsum). This is described by the chemical equation $CaSO_4 \ H_2O + H_2O = CaSO_4 \ 2H_2O + heat$. This is an exothermic reaction in which the powdered plaster of Paris becomes a rock-like mass.

Plaster bandages are available in a variety of widths (2-, 3-, 4-, 6-, and 8-inch wide rolls) and as splints (3 x 15 inches, 4 x 15 inches, and 5 x 30 inches). The setting time of the plaster is determined by the manufacturers and the temperature of the water into which it is dipped.

Fiberglass casting material has gained popularity in recent years. The cast tape is a rapidly curing fiberglass tape which sets in minutes.[2] The advantages of this material is that it is strong, lightweight, and waterproof. The major disadvantage of the material is that it requires skill to handle, is more difficult to mold, and is significantly more expensive than plaster. It is best used for long-term casts, and in patients who are particularly "hard" on casts. This type of material has little use in the acute injury setting where a cast will require a frequent change.

Most casts and splints are applied over a layer of cast padding with or without stockinette. Several types of padding are available including sheet cotton, Webril, and synthetic polypropolene (for fiberglass casts). This material is also available in a number of widths (2-, 3-, 4-, 5-, and 6-inch wide rolls). Padding is rolled onto the extremity to be casted, overlapping each turn by 50%. Particular attention must be paid to padding bony prominences such as the fibular head, the malleoli, the patella and the epicondyles of the humerus. Cast padding should be rolled onto the extremity such that it is free of wrinkles and folds. Care must also be taken not to "clump" padding over joints, specifically the dorsum of the ankle joint and the elbow crease.

Stockinette is not necessary for cast application. It does, however, improve the overall appearance of the finished product. In the patellar tendonbearing cast described by Sarmiento for the treatment of fractures of the tibia, the plaster is applied directly to a single layer of stockinette.

Splinting[2,4]

Splinting is a useful method of immobilization in the acute injury period. A satisfactory mold can be applied to the splint to hold the fracture alignment while the splint allows for swelling to occur without the development of ischemic contractures from the cast. The disadvantage of the splint is that the construct is not as stable as a circular cast, and the splint will loosen rapidly with time. Careful follow-up is necessary to prevent a loss of reduction when using a splint.

Plaster is the most commonly used splinting material. In most cases, splints will be converted to casts after the swelling has receded. In fractures, splints are applied over cast padding and held in place with bias cut stockinette or elastic bandages (Ace wrap). If Ace wraps are to be used to hold splints, care must be taken not to apply too much compression to the splint.

In the upper extremity, the sugar-tong splint gives excellent immobilization while allowing for significant swelling. A short-arm sugar-tong does incorporate the elbow. This primarily controls supination-pronation of the extremity. In fractures where flexion-extension of the elbow must be controlled, the sugar-tong can be reinforced above the elbow with an additional layer of plaster applied posteriorly with the elbow flexed 90 degrees.

In the lower extremity a posterior splint is formed by three sets of splints applied from toes to just distal to the knee. The splints are applied so as to not overlap anteriorly, and this allows for swelling. In fractures of the tibia where internal and external rotation must be controlled, the plaster splint is extended in all three planes (medial, lateral, and posterior) above the knee.

Radial and ulnar gutter splints are useful in maintaining wrist position in metacarpal fractures and carpal fractures. These splints consist of a single slab of splints applied with or without cast padding to the radial or ulnar aspects of the forearm. These splints can be fashioned to extend over the metacarpophalangeal joints. When the splints are extended onto the hand for the treatment of metacarpal fracture, care must be taken to obtain a satisfactory mold. If the slab is thick, the mold may not be adequate to maintain the reduction.

Malleable aluminum splints are available in several sizes. They can be contoured by hand and cut with tin snips to the appropriate size. These splints are useful in phalangeal fractures, dislocations, and volar plate injuries. They are also useful for the closed treatment of mallet finger.

Casting[2,4]

The basic rule of casting is to immobilize a joint above and below the level of a fracture. This is necessary to give rotational stability of the fracture. Many joints will stiffen with prolonged immobilization despite appropriate physical therapy after cast removal. For example, immobilization of the metacarpophalangeal joints in extension for periods as short as three weeks can result in loss of range of motion. If the metacarpophalangeal joints must be immobilized for extended periods, they should be immobilized in 90 degrees of flexion if possible. Flexion maintains the length of the collateral ligaments and allows for recovery of range of motion after immobilization.

Upper extremity casting can be divided into long- and short-arm casts. Short-arm casts are used for metacarpal fractures and carpal fractures acutely; and they are used for protection of distal radius fractures during the late phases of healing. Long-arm casts are used for fractures of the ulna, radius and distal humerus. In addition, a lightweight long-arm cast can be used with a sling for the treatment of midshaft humerus fractures.

Lower extremity casts are divided into three general types, short-leg (SLC [below-knee]), long-leg (LLC [above-knee]), and patellar tendonbearing (PTB). The SLC protects the ankle but does not control rotation of the tibia. A well-molded PTB or LLC will control lower leg rotation.

The development of the cast boot has simplified the conversion of non-weightbearing casts to walking casts. The cast boot allows for better weight distribution over a greater surface area than the rubber walking heel. Casts used for weightbearing are subjected to greater stress than nonweightbearing casts, and these casts warrant reinforcement over the heel, ankle, and knee.

Casting and Splinting Techniques[2,4]

Prior to the reduction of a fracture or application of a splint or cast, a full examination of the extremity must be made. This examination should include a full neurovascular assessment, a description of the appearance of the extremity, a grading of the amount of swelling, and the skin condition. The range of motion of all joints to be immobilized should be documented.

All materials for the cast or splint should be assembled before a reduction is attempted or application is begun. This should include sufficient padding, casting material, stockinette, and bias wrap and tape, if needed. A bucket of water should be available for dipping the casting material. Water should be changed after each application as the temperature and residual plaster in the water will alter setting time. The water temperature should be lukewarm - hot water will speed setting time, but such an exothermic reaction can cause skin burns.

All splints and casts require molding. Fracture reductions are maintained with three point fixation. A rule of thumb for molding of a cast is that the cast should look like the extremity that was casted. Specific molds should be made about the wrist and hand to ensure full range of motion of nonimmobilized digits. The epicondyles of the humerus should be molded as well as the triceps in long-arm casts. In lower extremity casts, the arch of the foot, malleoli, tendo-Achilles, and anterior crest of the tibia should be molded. The patella, femoral condyles and quadriceps must be molded to obtain a well-fitting long-leg cast.

Upper Extremity Splints[1,2,4]

Sugar-tong Splints[1]: The arm is padded from the metacarpophalangeal joints to above the elbow with cast padding. The splint is a continuous slab of plaster extending from the distal palmar crease to the elbow and over the dorsal surface of the hand to end over the dorsum of the metacarpophalangeal joints. Unroll a three- or four-inch roll of plaster to make a single slab which will reach the above distance. Since the injured extremity is usually painful, it is wise to measure the desired length by using a pattern on the opposite or uninjured limb. To obtain the desired thickness (7-10 thicknesses), often two or three rolls of plaster are necessary. While the patient's arm is held in the desired position by an assistant, the plaster slab is dipped and applied to the extremity, and held on with a layer of elastic bandage or bias cut stockinette. The splint is molded to the extremity, and held until it is set (Fig. 7-1). In the upper extremity, particular attention must be paid to the hand to avoid contractures (especially extension contractures of the MCPJ, adduction contractures of the thumb, and flexion contractures of the wrist and PIPJ). Once the cast has set, the patient should be checked to ensure that full motion of the hand is present. In distal radius (Colles') fractures, the sugar-tong may be extended onto the upper arm with an additional slab of plaster. This minimizes motion of the elbow.

Coaptation Splints[1]: This splint is useful for the immobilization of fractures of the humerus. It is a sugar-tong splint of the upper extremity. The patient's arm is padded from shoulder to below-the-elbow. A single splint is again constructed from rolls of plaster. The splint should extend from the above the acromion, over the lateral aspect of the arm to the elbow, and incorporating the elbow, it should extend into the axilla. This splint should also be 7-12 thicknesses of plaster. It is applied over the padding and wrapped into place with bias cut. When using this splint, the shoulder is placed into adduction and internal rotation. The forearm is immobilized with a commercially available shoulder immobilizer or it is held to the trunk with a sling and swathe.

Ulnar Gutter Splints: Ulnar gutter splints are useful for the treatment of night stick fractures of the ulna and fractures of the neck of the fourth and fifth metacarpals (boxer's fractures). The mold of this splint is important to obtain immobilization. If the forearm and hand are heavily padded, the gutter will not encompass enough of the ulna and hypothenar eminence to control motion and maintain a reduction. This splint consists of a single slab of plaster (5-8 thick) applied over a lightly padded forearm and hand. Care should be taken not to allow padding to gather in the folds of the fingers. This splint should be wrapped snugly with a bias stockinette and followed closely for loosening. (Bias-cut stockinette will loosen within 24 hours.)

Aluminum Splints: These splints are used to immobilize phalangeal fractures, as well as volar plate injuries at the PIP joints. The PIP joint should be immobilized in 10 degrees of flexion or less to maintain a full range of motion. (The accessory collateral ligaments tighten with the PIPJ held in flexion.) These splints can also be incorporated into casts and dorsal splints to obtain immobilization of metacarpal fractures. When incorporating the MCP joint in these splints, care must be taken to immobilize the MCPJ in 60-90 degrees of flexion, to avoid extension contractures from shortening of the collateral ligaments.

Lower Extremity Splints[1,2,4]

Posterior Splints: This splint immobilizes the ankle. It has applications for isolated fibula fractures, metatarsal fractures, and ankle sprains. It should be noted that ankle fractures require long-leg immobilization in order to control rotation. This will be a long leg cast eventually, but initially a long-leg splint may be used.

These splints can be applied without assistance if the patient is able to cooperate. The patient should be posititioned in the prone position with the knee flexed 90 degrees. Most patients can maintain this position without difficulty, and the splint can be easily applied.

The lower extremity is padded from toe to knee with additional padding being placed over the malleoli and the fibular head. In adults, the splint can be easily constructed from three sets of 5 x 30-inch splints (5-10 thicknesses each). These splints are applied over the padding. The medial slab begins 2-4 cm below the medial joint line of the knee, and extends distally to encompass the heel, and the lateral malleolus. The lateral slab is applied at the level of the fibular head, and extends distally to overlap the medial slab at the heel. This forms a

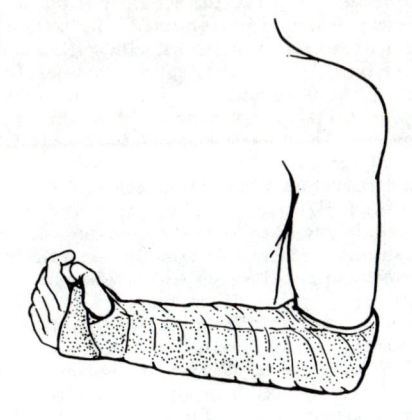

Fig. 7-1

Sugar-tong Splint

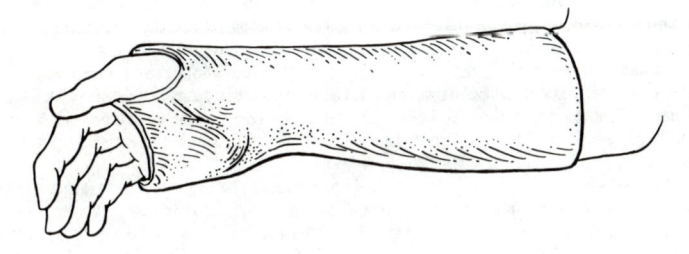

Fig. 7-2

Short-arm Cast

sugar-tong around the ankle. The splint is completed by bringing a third slab from just distal to the knee over the heel and out over the toes. Excess material is folded back on itself to form a footplate. The splint is wrapped into place with bias cut stockinette. When wrapping, do not allow the plaster to overlap over the anterior aspect of the leg. The splint is completed by molding the ankle into neutral. The suggested thicknesses are 10-thick for the posterior slab, and 5-thick for the medial and lateral slabs.

Long-leg Posterior Splints: This splint is useful for the treatment of ankle fractures or tibia fractures where severe swelling is expected. The posterior splint is not as stable a construct as a bivalved or split cast, but it allows for greater swelling without the development of ischemic contracture. A long-leg splint is applied in the same fashion as a short-leg splint initially, and then it is extended above the knee with additional plaster slabs placed along the medial, lateral, and posterior aspects of the thigh. In addition to the mold of the splint at the malleolus, the splint can be molded at the thigh.

Upper Extremity Casts[2,4]

Short-arm Cast: The short-arm cast is applied over a single layer of cast padding. It extends from just proximal to the distal palmar crease to just distal to the elbow. In adults, rolls of 3- and 4-inch plaster allow for easy application and a good finish. The cast is most easily applied with the patient lying supine with the shoulder abducted 90 degrees, elbow flexed 90 degrees, and the hand directed toward the ceiling. In this position, the short-arm cast can be applied without assistance if the patient is able to cooperate. Plaster is rolled onto the extremity beginning at the hand. Several turns are taken through the palm. The plaster should be gathered through the web space so as not to interfere with thumb motion. The cast is then extended down the forearm to stop just distal to the elbow. Since a cross-section of the forearm has an oval or elliptical configuration, the cast should be molded in this manner rather than round or circular. This can be acheived by molding with the flat of both palms and gently pressing against the radius and ulna to spread the interosseus membrane. The cast should not interfere with elbow flexion or extension, although it should extend as far proximally as the range of motion will permit.

After the cast has set, the patient should have 90 degrees of flexion at the metacarpophalangeal joints. The thumb should have full extension and be able to oppose with the little finger. If the cast limits this motion it should be trimmed with a cast knife or power saw (Fig. 7-2).

Thumb Spica Cast: This modification of the short- or long-arm cast is used for scaphoid fractures, the immobilization of Bennett's fractures (fractures of the base the first metacarpal), and for use in some thumb phalangeal fractures. This cast extends to the distal part of the thumb, its exact extent depending on fracture location and the physician's experience and judgment. It should always immobilize the MCPJ of the thumb, and may be extended distal to the thumb IPJ. The difficulty with this cast is to obtain adequate thicknesses of plaster to immobilize the thumb without wadding cast material into the palm and inhibiting motion of the MCP joints of the other digits. One method is to use 2- or 3-inch splints one thickness at a time, and apply them longitudinally and circumferentially to the thumb. The splints need only be long enough to extend to the base of the wrist where they can be captured with a roll of plaster.

Long-arm Cast: The long-arm cast is an extension of the short-arm cast and it is used when forearm rotation must be controlled. The cast is applied to the forearm and arm over a layer of plaster and stockinette. Sufficient padding must be applied about the elbow to protect the ulnar nerve as it crosses the elbow over its posteromedical border in the ulnar groove of humerus.

While larger rolls of plaster can be used to apply casts to the arm (i.e., 6-inch rolls), 4-inch rolls are satisfactory. In the upper arm and thigh there is enough soft tissue present that the cast material can be "pulled" to obtain a well-fitting snug cast. In applying casts to the foot, ankle, leg, and forearm, plaster should be pushed onto the extremity and never stretched or "pulled."

The long-arm cast then is applied by first applying a short-arm cast and then extending it above the elbow. To reinforce the elbow, 3 x 15- or 4 x 15-inch splints can be placed on the medial, lateral and posterior sides. This creates a strong cast at the elbow without the need for additional circumferential layers of plaster. Attention must be paid to not gather cast padding in the elbow crease, which is constricting and can cause pressure problems. Gathering of the plaster in the elbow joint can be avoided by loosely taking a figure-8 turn around the elbow.

Finally the cast is then molded with attention paid to mold the upper arm over the humeral condyles and biceps muscle. A triangular mold of the upper arm can be made by resting the upper arm on a flat surface, while manually molding above the humeral condyles. Although it is possible to apply this cast without assistance, the patients find it difficult to maintain their elbow at 90 degrees while the plaster is setting (Fig. 7-3).

Hanging Arm Casts: This cast is a special application of the long-arm cast used to immobilize humeral shaft fractures. This cast is merely a lightweight long-arm cast applied from a point two-inches proximal to the fracture site on the humerus. The arm is held reduced by a sling built into the cast at the wrist. By adjusting the length of the rope, and the place on the cast where the rope is attached (on the volar or dorsal aspect of the wrist), a reduction can be achieved and maintained. One difficulty with this cast is that the patient must remain in an upright position until the fracture has healed (this includes sleeping in a chair).

The cast is applied in standard fashion, although the padding and casting material used must be kept to minimum to prevent distraction of the fracture by the weight of the cast. A piece of coat hanger wire can be affixed to the cast at the wrist, to afford an easy attachment point for the sling which can be manipulated. This is one cast where fiberglass might be used in the acute situation to maintain a low-weight construct. A practical approach to humeral

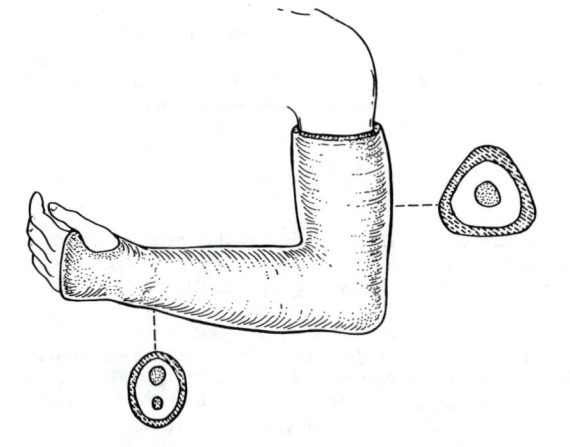

Fig. 7-3

Long-arm Cast

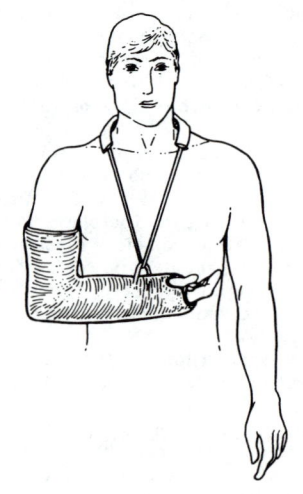

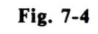

Fig. 7-4

Hanging Cast

shaft fractures is to maintain the patient in a coaptation splint for 7-10 days after the injury until the swelling has subsided, and then to apply a fiberglass hanging arm cast or commercially available coaptation splint (Fig. 7-4).

Lower Extremity Casts[2,4]

Short-leg Casts: The short-leg cast is the mainstay for all ankle injuries. It can be used for the stabilization of acute ankle instabilities, and it can be used as a protective cast when weightbearing on partially healed fractures of the ankle and tibia/fibula.

The short-leg cast is applied over a single layer of cast padding. Before applying plaster, make certain that the malleoli, heel and fibular head are well padded. When applying the casting material, make certain that enough material has been applied to the heel. If the cast is to be used for weightbearing, then three or four 4 x 15 splints applied anteriorly, medially and laterally around the ankle will reinforce the cast at the most common site of breakdown. A common error made is not to carry the cast high enough on the leg, and it will subsequently slip down on the ankle. The cast should be carried distal to the fibular head. A snug fitting cast can be obtained by loosely taking several figure-8 turns around the proximal gastrocsoleus to lock in the muscle belly and prevent the cast from slipping. (Do not "pull" or stretch the plaster.) After the first two rolls of plaster have been applied, the foot and ankle should be molded. If not holding an acute reduction of a fracture, the ankle should be molded in the neutral position (90 degrees to the lower leg). If the cast is to be used for weightbearing, gait will be improved by molding the ankle into slight dorsiflexion (5-10 degrees).

Additional plaster should be applied to the sole of the cast when it is to be used for weightbearing. A footplate which covers the heel and extends past the ends of the toes is easily fashioned out of 4 x 15 splints and affixed to the cast with a roll of plaster. When affixing the footplate, be sure to take several turns longitudinally around the footplate to completely lock it onto the cast (Fig. 7-5).

When the cast is complete, the dorsum of the foot should be trimmed so that all toes are visible. Trimming can be done with a cast knife, scalpel, or oscillating saw. If care is taken while applying the footplate excessive trimming is not necessary.

Long-leg Cast: Most applications of the long-leg cast are for the closed treatment of tibia fractures or ankle fractures. The leg is padded in the usual fashion. Because the thigh has more fat tissue, the cast padding should be wrapped snugly around the thigh. A short-leg cast is applied as described, and the application is continued above the knee. The leg must be held by an assistant in the desired amount of knee flexion until the plaster has set. In the application of the casting material, the plaster may be pulled taut around the upper thigh only to obtain a snug fit. The cast should be carried to within inches of the

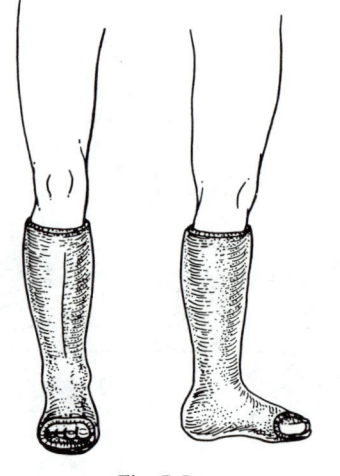

Fig. 7-5

Short-leg Cast

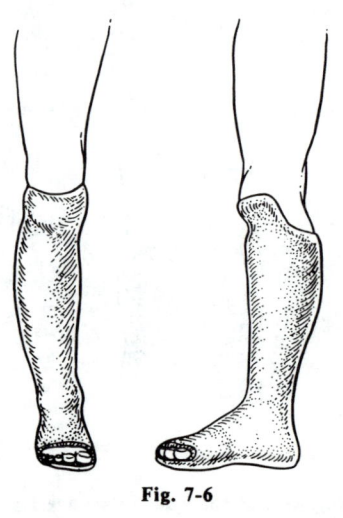

Fig. 7-6

Patellar-tendon Bearing (PTB) Cast

Long Leg Cast (LLC)

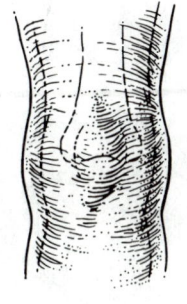

Molding the knee joint
in a LLC

Fig. 7-7

Molding Around the Knee in a Long-leg Cast

groin on the medial side. Splints should be used to reinforce the knee, and these are best applied medially, laterally, and anteriorly. In the application of the long-leg cast, six inch plaster rolls should be used above the ankle as this will allow for a faster application and a better finish (Fig. 7-7).

The mold of the thigh and knee are crucial to the efficacy of this cast. The cast must be molded around the condyles of the femur so as not to slide down the leg. A quadrilateral thigh mold is applied manually by placing the heels of the palms just above the knee on the medial and lateral sides. With pressure, the cast will take on a rectangular configuration. When the patient ambulates, the cast will be carried by the supracondylar mold (Fig. 7-7).

Patellar-tendon bearing Cast: This cast was first developed by Sarmiento for the treatment of tibia fractures without immobilizing the knee. Sarmiento's initial description calls for no cast padding to be used, with the cast material to be applied directly onto stockinette. The patellar-tendon bearing cast is frequently used to allow early ambulation; however, cast padding is recommended in the application of the casts.

This cast is essentially applied as a long-leg cast with the knee flexed at 30-45 degrees, and the ankle in neutral. Extra material must be applied over the condyles laterally and medially, as well as over the patellar tendon anteriorly. The cast is well molded around the proximal tibial flare, and the patellar tendon is molded horizontally. After the plaster has set, the cast is cut down to allow for flexion at the knee while the condylar "wings" prevent rotation, and the patella tendon and proximal medial tibial flare bear a majority of the weight (Fig. 7-6).

Spica Casts:[3] Body casts are rarely used for the immobilization of fractures of the upper extremity. Lower extremity spica casts are used for a number of applications which include: femoral shaft fractures and to maintain a hip reduced after dislocation and closed reduction (currently most commonly seen in dislocated total hip arthroplasties). The casts are also used in congenital hip dislocations to maintain the child's hips in abduction and flexion.

This cast requires several assistants to apply expeditiously and correctly. The patient can either be placed on a spica table, or if the patient can stand, the cast can be applied with the patient standing. Stockinette should be applied over the entire surface to be casted. Depending on the intention of the cast, the cast can include one thigh (single pantaloon), two thighs (pantaloon), one entire leg (single-hip spica), and both legs (double-hip spica).

Padding should consist of not only a layer of cast padding, but felt strips should be applied to prominences. These areas include the iliac crests, the spine, and the costal margins. Additional felt should be placed at the superior and inferior aspects of the cast for additional comfort, especially if the patient is to be ambulating.

The cast is applied circumferentially with 6- or 8-inch rolls of cast material. After a layer of cast material is applied, the remainder of the cast consists of 5 x 30-inch splints which are applied in layers of 3-5 thicknesses. When applying the splints, particular attention must be paid to the area where the cast crosses the hip joint (intern's angle). This is the area most susceptible to breakdown from stress as the cast is not supported circumferentially at that point.

When the cast has set, it can be trimmed. A circular hole should be made in the abdomen for feeding, and the cast should be trimmed around the perineal area. Finally, when the cast has dried completely, small areas of irritation can be padded with moleskin for comfort. An example of a spica cast is shown in Fig. 7-8.

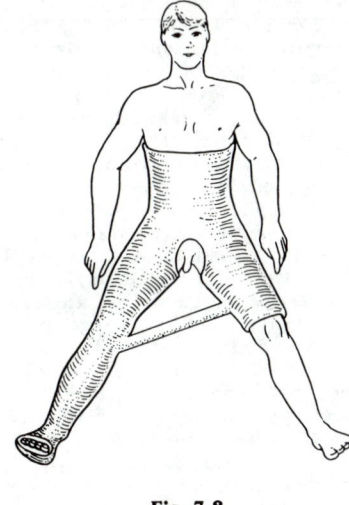

Fig. 7-8

Hip Spica Cast

References

1.   Charnley JA. *The Closed Treatment of Common Fractures.* Edinburgh: Churchill-Livingstone, 1972.
2.   Lewis RC Jr. *Handbook of Traction, Casting, and Splinting Techniques.* Philadelphia: J. B. Lippincott, 1972.
3.   Rockwood CA, Green DP. *Fractures In Adults (Volume 1).* 2nd edition. Philadelphia: J. B. Lippincott, 1984.
4.   Schneider FR. *Handbook for the Orthopaedic Assistant.* St. Louis: C. V. Mosby, 1976.

Chapter 8

Traction Techniques

With the increasing use of primary internal fixation and the improvements in external fixation systems, there has been a decrease in the use of traction. Traction, however, remains a useful option in adult fracture management. Rarely, traction is used as the definitive treatment of adult fractures, but it is useful if there is a delay in taking the patient to the operating room.

In the pediatric population, traction is still widely employed in the treatment of femur fractures in the preadolescent age group, in the treatment of congenital hip dislocation, and in treating Legg-Calvé-Perthes disease. In this population, traction is usually the initial treatment and is followed by plaster immobilization or bracing.

The purpose of traction in the treatment of fractures is to obtain satisfactory alignment of the fracture. This is performed by aligning the distal fragment with the proximal fragment through the use of continuous applied distraction. The deforming forces acting across the fracture must be known so the traction can be positioned to overcome these forces. For instance, in a distal femur fracture, the distal fragment is flexed by the gastrocnemius and pulled medially by the adductors. When a patient with this fracture is placed in traction, the knee is flexed to remove the effect of the gastrocnemius, and traction on the tibial pin would be placed such that the lower leg is slightly abducted. To adequately use traction, the physician must understand the force vectors applied by the traction apparatus.

TRACTION REQUIRES CONSTANT VIGILANCE by the health care team. In the course of moving patients for linen changes or imaging studies, the traction will often be disconnected or malaligned. A responsible member of the team must check the patient at least daily to assess the adequacy of the traction. Frequent radiographs must be obtained to insure the adequacy of the reduction.

This chapter is intended as an introduction to the many types of traction. Traction should never be applied without the supervision of an experienced physician. The patient can be significantly harmed by the misuse of traction with complications including neurovascular injury. When in doubt about the use or application of traction, consult someone who is experienced IMMEDIATELY.

Traction Setup

Before instituting traction, the bed must be fitted with the proper equipment. This usually includes an overhead frame with multiple outrigger bars for the attachment of pulleys. The overhead frame is usually provided with a trapeze handle so the patient may move in bed. For any patient who is unconscious or who will be treated for an extended period of time in bed, the mattress of the bed should be supplemented with an egg crate or water mattress for the prevention of decubitus ulcers. In addition, special air mattresses and rotation beds exist for patients who will be recumbent for long periods of time. Their use should be considered in any patient such as this who will be at high risk for the formation of decubiti.

Types of Traction[1,2]

Traction can be divided into two general types by the method of application of the force - skin or skeletal. In skin traction the pull of the weights is applied to the skin. This type of traction limits the amount of force that can be applied before injury to the skin will occur. Skin is very susceptible to shear forces and all skin traction should be removed and reapplied whenever the patient has a complaint, or every 48 hours. Skin traction does not allow for precise rotational control of fractures. Therefore, the use of skin traction is limited to applications where the maximum weight is less than 7 lbs and the traction must not maintain precise rotational control.

Skeletal traction uses pins placed into or through bone to apply the traction force. The advantages of this system are that greater forces can be applied, the traction bow affords good rotational control, and the traction can be maintained for a long period of time (8-12 weeks). The disadvantages of skeletal traction are related to the pins. Pins can pull out, and pin tracts can become infected. Occasionally, pin tract infections can lead to osteomyelitis. There is also some risk of neurovascular injury in the placement of the pins. In the adolescent population, the pin can be improperly placed into the physis and cause a growth disturbance. Placement of traction pins is discussed in Chapter Five (*Orthopaedic Emergencies and Emergency Room Techniques*).

Specific Types of Traction

Buck's Traction:[1,2,3,4] Buck's traction is really a misnomer. The purpose of Buck's traction is to maintain the leg in extension. This traction is most commonly used in the temporary treatment of intertrochanteric, and femoral neck fractures. The traction pulls the hip and knee into extension in order to make the patient comfortable until more definitive fixation can be performed. The traction does not serve to reduce or align the fracture; it merely improves the pain.

The traction is applied to the leg by a foam boot which fits the foot and calf. This boot is then connected to a traction rope and weight pan as shown in Fig. 8-1. This is a skin traction system, and the traction boot must be removed frequently to check the condition of the skin.

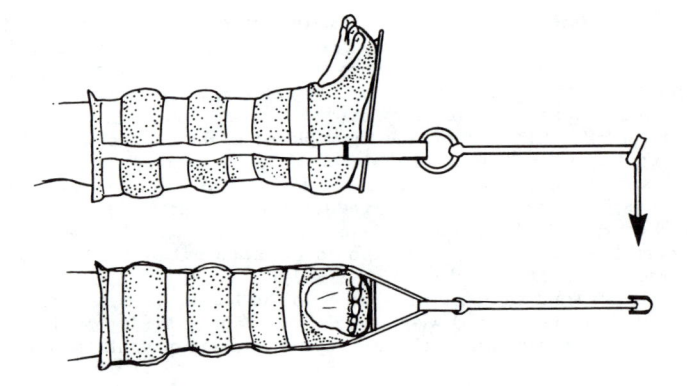

Fig. 8-1

Buck's Traction

Bryant's Traction:[1,2,3,4] Bryant's traction is used in the first stage of the reduction of a dislocated hip in the younger patient with congenital dislocation of the hip (3-18 months). The goal of traction in congenital dislocated hips (CDH) is to gently bring the femoral head into alignment with the triradiate cartilage of the developing acetabulum. Because the hip in CDH may have been dislocated for some time, the muscles and soft tissues are contracted around the hip joint. Prereduction traction allows gentle reduction of the femoral head and lessens the risk of avascular necrosis of the femoral head as a complication of overzealous reduction maneuvers.

The traction is a skin traction which consists of felt or moleskin strips applied to the lower extremities and held in place with elastic wraps. The felt strips are connected to a traction cord which is run overhead to the edge of the bed. This is shown in Fig. 8-2.

The hips are maintained in 90 degrees of flexion and 30 degrees of abduction. Some knee flexion is permitted to relax the hamstrings. The amount of weight applied is just enough to lift the buttocks off the bed or a maximum of 5 lbs. If additional traction is necessary, Russell's or split-Russell's traction may be used.

Bryant's traction is a dangerous method of traction that can cause vascular compromise to the lower leg. Because of this, it is absolutely contraindicated in children over six months of age, who are at even higher risk for this complication. In addition, even in infants, the vascular status of the leg must be checked several times daily during the duration of application of Bryant's traction.

Split-Russell's:[1,2,3] Split-Russell's traction can be used in some femur fractures as well as in hip traction for patients with Legg-Calvé-Perthes disease, or a older patient with CDH. This system is usually employed when the patient is too large or old for Bryant's traction. The application of force in two planes increases the resultant force vector on the hip.

In split-Russell's traction, the leg is placed in Buck's traction, and a knee sling is applied to the knee and proximal tibia with an upward force. This traction is shown in Fig. 8-3. When this traction is used for CDH, the hips are kept moderately flexed (60 degrees), abducted 30-40 degrees, and the knees are flexed 60 degrees. If this traction is being used for long-term treatment of Legg-Calvé-Perthes disease, the patient should be taken out of traction for brief periods each day to examine the skin.

Russell's traction applies all forces to the leg in the same direction but uses a single traction cord and weight. This tends to keep the leg in slightly more extension. These systems are rarely used in the treatment of adult fractures.

90/90 Upper Arm Traction and Side-arm Traction:[2,3,4] 90/90 and side-arm tractions are used to treat fractures of the humerus. These systems can be used with an olecranon pin or skin traction. The olecranon pin must be placed carefully to avoid the ulnar nerve on the medial side of the elbow.

The purpose of 90/90 and side-arm traction is to obtain longitudinal traction of the humerus and support the forearm in the proper rotation. When

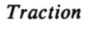

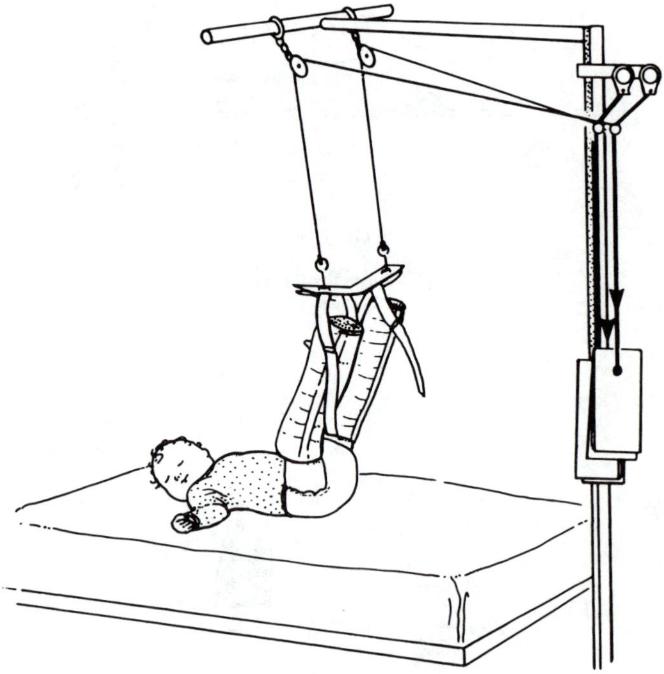

Fig. 8-2

Bryant's Traction

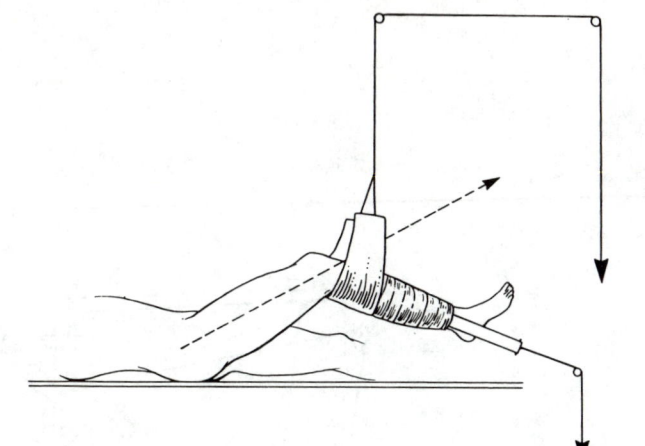

Fig. 8-3

Split-Russell's Traction

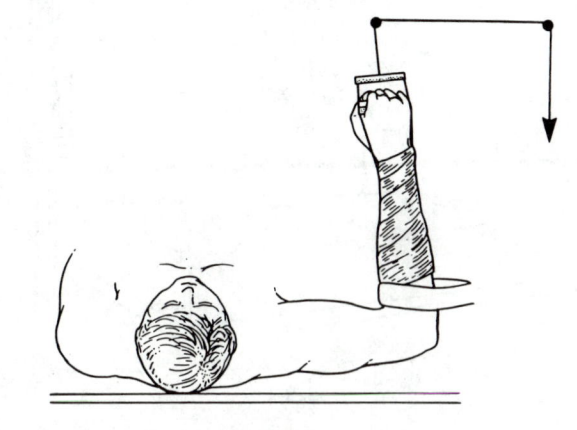

Fig. 8-4

Side-arm Skin Traction

treated in this fashion, the humerus will unite quickly even in the adult patient, and once early union has been obtained, the patient can be converted to another form of immobilization which is less confining.

In side-arm traction, skin traction or olecranon pin traction is placed on the arm with the patient supine in bed, and the arm abducted 90 degrees. This traction pulls perpendicular to the long axis of the body. Additional skin traction is applied to the forearm with the elbow flexed 90 degrees and the wrist in neutral. The forearm traction supports the weight of the forearm perpendicular to the coronal plane of the body. This is shown in Fig. 8-4.

In 90/90 traction, the arm traction is placed directly overhead with the shoulder positioned in 90 degrees of forward flexion. The forearm is then positioned in the same plane as the bed and is supported by a sling.

90/90 Femoral Traction:[1,2,3] 90/90 femoral traction is a form of traction devised specifically for the management of subtrochanteric fractures in adults. In addition, it can be used to manage some high femoral shaft fractures in children. In 90/90 femoral traction, a pin is placed through the distal femur. The leg is then suspended by skeletal traction through this pin such that the femur is flexed 90 degrees at the hip. The knee is also flexed 90 degrees, hence the name 90/90 traction. Usually, the lower leg is attached to a splint or a Buck's traction boot, and this is attached to a light weight brought over the foot end of the bed. This prevents rotation of the leg at the hip and provides for greater fracture stability and patient comfort (Fig. 8-5).

90/90 traction is effective in subtrochanteric fractures because, by flexing the hip 90 degrees, the distal fracture fragments are made to align with the proximal fragment which is usually flexed acutely by the pull of the iliopsoas.

Balanced Skeletal Traction:[1,2,3,4] Balanced skeletal traction is most commonly used in the temporary treatment of femur fractures. This traction uses a skeletal traction pin placed in the proximal tibia or distal femur connected to a traction bow. The use of traction pins allows for greater forces to be applied for fracture reduction. The remainder of the leg is then supported on a splint or frame which is well padded. The amount of knee flexion can be varied to assist in the reduction of the fracture when the gastrocnemius is a major deforming factor. In addition, the splint and leg can be abducted to compensate for the deforming force of the adductors.

Traction pins should be carefully placed with the surgeon conscious of the nearby neurovascular structures. If a more definitive treatment of the femur fracture is planned, a tibial pin should be placed rather than femoral pins, as the femoral pin will theoretically contaminate the intramedullary canal. Before the tibial pin is placed, an accurate examination of the knee must be made to insure its stability. <u>DO NOT APPLY TRACTION THROUGH AN UNSTABLE KNEE!</u>

The Thomas splint with Pearson attachment is the most common splint system used in balanced skeletal traction. In using this splint, a common mistake is the selection of too large a splint for the patient. Subsequently, the Pearson attachment is well below the knee. This traction is demonstrated in Fig. 8-7.

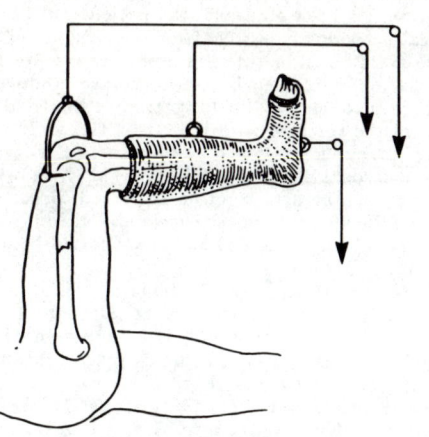

Fig. 8-5

90/90 Traction

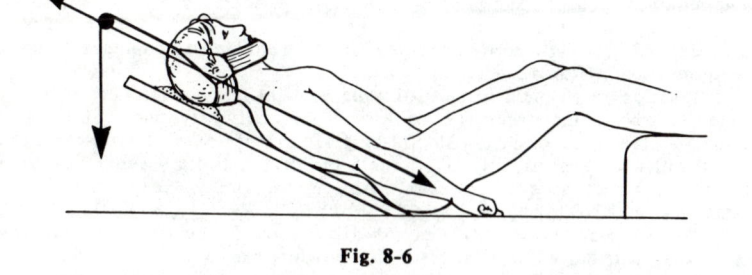

Fig. 8-6

Cervical Traction

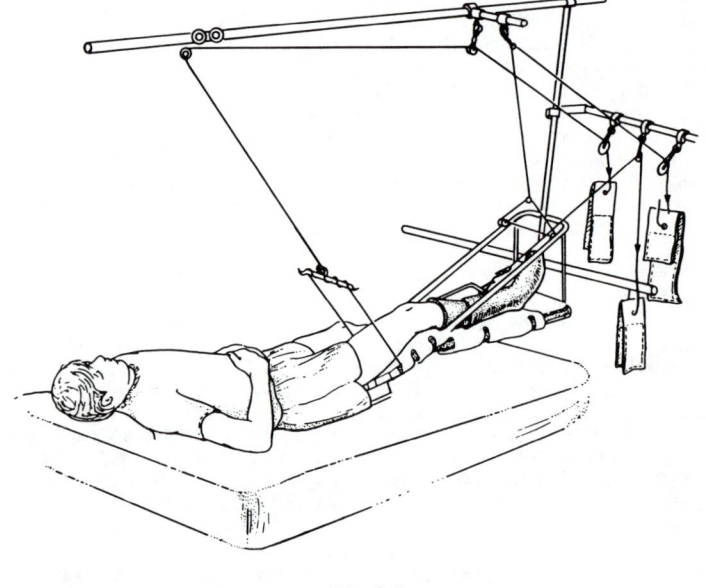

Fig. 8-7

Balanced Skeletal Traction

Cervical Traction: Cervical traction is used in the conservative treatment of cervical spondylosis. The purpose is to allow for some decompression of the facet joints, and temporary relief of pain. This is usually prescribed as a home program where the patient uses the traction intermittently several times per day.

Cervical traction is available in two configurations: 1) traction applied with the patient sitting; and 2) traction applied with the patient in the supine position. The patient uses a head halter which runs beneath the chin and occiput and is then connected to a spreader bar. Weight is then applied for traction as shown in Fig. 8-6. In the sitting position, 12-15 lbs of traction are used, and in the supine position 5-7 lbs are applied.

Halo and Gardner-Wells Tong Traction:[1,2,3,4] This form of traction is used in the reduction and stabilization of cervical spine fractures. Only experienced physicians should apply or adjust this traction. Many cervical fractures can be reduced by closed traction. This is facilitated by the application of either Gardner-Wells tongs or the halo ring. When the halo ring is used in fracture reduction, the pins must be tightened to 6 kg-cm prior to the application of traction. With the Gardner-Wells tongs, longitudinal traction can be applied; however, rotation can be difficult to control. The halo ring gives better rotational control of the head.

With these devices applied, traction is then obtained by connecting the tongs or ring to a traction cord at the head of the bed. To obtain direct longitudinal traction, some hospital beds will require an additional mattress to allow the traction cord to clear the head of the bed. The amount of flexion and extension of the cervical spine is controlled by the amount of elevation of the head of the bed. Any movement of the bed will change the direction of the traction. All electric beds should be turned off once they are in the desired position.

Traction can then be applied gradually. The general rule of thumb is that 10 lbs of weight should be used to overcome the weight of the head, and an additional 5 lbs for each level of the cervical spine through which traction need be applied. For instance, in a fracture or dislocation at the C-5 level, 35 lbs of weight would be used - 10 lbs for the head, and 25 lbs to overcome the pull of the five levels of the cervical spine. It is usually recommended to start by applying about 20 lbs of traction initially and then increase it in 5-lb increments. **AFTER THE INITIAL ADDITION OF WEIGHT AND AFTER ANY CHANGE IN THE TRACTION OR WEIGHT, THE POSITION OF THE CERVICAL FRACTURE SHOULD BE IMMEDIATELY CHECKED WITH A LATERAL VIEW OF THE CERVICAL SPINE. CAREFUL DOCUMENTATION OF THE NEUROLOGIC STATUS OF THE PATIENT IS MANDATORY AFTER EACH CHANGE IN WEIGHT OR POSITION. ANY DETERIORATION IN NEUROLOGIC STATUS IS AN INDICATION TO IMMEDIATELY RETURN TO THE PREVIOUS LEVEL OR POSITION OF TRACTION.** The patient must be maintained in an intensive care setting while the fracture is being reduced.

If the halo ring is employed in the reduction, the halo jacket can be applied to stabilize the cervical spine after the reduced position is achieved.

References

1. Lewis RC Jr. *Handbook of Traction, Casting, and Splinting Techniques.* Philadelphia: J. B. Lippincott, 1977.
2. Schmeisser G Jr. *A Clinical Manual of Orthopaedic Traction Techniques.* Philadelphia: W. B. Saunders, 1963.
3. Schneider FR. *Handbook for the Orthopaedic Assistant.* 2nd edition. St. Louis: C. V. Mosby, 1976.
4. *The Traction Handbook.* Warsaw, Indiana: Zimmer, 1980.

Chapter 9

Perioperative Orthopaedic Care

Preoperative Evaluation and Screening

The orthopaedic surgical candidate can vary from a debilitated elderly person with a hip fracture and multiple medical problems to a robust adolescent football player with a knee injury. Preoperative evaluation of both patients is important, but it must be individualized. Obviously, the preoperative evaluation begins with a thorough history and physical examination. After this is completed, specific laboratory studies are also obtained, as suggested by the history and physical examination.

The preoperative evaluation for orthopaedic surgery usually includes, but is not limited to, the following:[24]

> Vital signs (temperature, BP, pulse)
> History
> Physical examination
> Complete blood count
> Serum chemistries
> Coagulation studies
> Urinalysis
> Chest radiograph
> Electrocardiogram

Although this is a standard protocol, the importance of evaluating each patient individually can be seen when analyzing the two patients mentioned above. The football player probably does not need all these studies, while the older person with a hip fracture may need several more.

Vital signs must be evaluated on all patients prior to any surgical procedure. If there is any abnormality, it should be studied further with the appropriate tests. This might include multiple cultures for a fever work-up, an EKG for an abnormal pulse, and evaluation of volume status for an abnormal blood pressure. An elevated temperature suggesting an occult infection will often cause the anaesthesiologist to balk at spinal or epidural anaesthesia. However, realistically, elective surgery should not be performed if the patient has an elevated temperature.

The six lab studies mentioned above are performed for specific reasons. The complete blood count should evaluate the hematocrit/hemoglobin (to ensure adequate oxygen carrying capacity during anaesthesia), the white blood cell count (to check for occult infections), and platelet count (to ensure adequate hemostasis).

Chemistries usually include Na^+, K^+, Cl^-, CO_2, BUN, glucose, and creatinine. Each is important and should be carefully evaluated. A complete description of the evaluation is beyond the scope of this text, but the Na^+, Cl^-, BUN, and creatinine can yield important clues as to the volume status of the patient. The K^+ is quite important, as hypo- or hyperkalemia during general anaesthesia can predispose to cardiac arrhythmias. The BUN and creatinine are used to evaluate renal function as well as volume status. The serum glucose is most important in patients with diabetes, and occasionally a patient will be discovered to be hyperglycemic on his preoperative evaluation with no previous knowledge of this condition.

Coagulation studies (PT, PTT) are usually ordered on major orthopaedic procedures such as total joint replacements, major fracture work, or spinal fusions and instrumentations. The hematology literature states that this is rarely indicated. The most important indicator of a bleeding diathesis is a past history of a bleeding tendency - bleeding after dental work, easy bruising, excessive menstrual flow in females. Also important would be a family history of a bleeding tendency.[6] In patients with either of these tendencies, the coagulation studies are indicated. Otherwise, it is probably not a cost-effective test. The reason that orthopaedists tend to order coagulation studies is because of the great amount of bleeding that occurs from exposed cancellous bone. There is no effective way to obtain complete mechanical hemostasis in these procedures; thus, the tests are usually ordered as a precaution.

The urinalysis is examined to preclude a urinary tract infection or renal problems. Infections can be catastrophic in elective cases where an implant will be used (total joints, or internal fixation of fractures). If a urinary tract infection is present, it must be treated preoperatively with an appropriate antibiotic. If the infection is severe, an elective total joint replacement may be better delayed until the infection is cleared. In nontrauma patients, the urinalysis is of minimal importance to the anaesthesiologist as long as renal function can be shown to be adequate by the chemistries and urine output. Consequently, emergency surgery should not be delayed because this study has not yet been completed.

The chest radiograph is examined to check for signs of cardiopulmonary pathology. However, a good physical examination of the chest and obtaining a detailed history about cardiopulmonary problems is far more cost-effective. As a result, this test does not need to be ordered in relatively young (under age 40), healthy patients.

The electrocardiogram (EKG) is another study that can usually be omitted in the young, healthy patient with a regular pulse and normal cardiac examination. A good history and physical examination will indicate any patients in this category who need an EKG to evaluate their heart further.

You will note from the above discussion that the healthy, adolescent football player probably only needs two of the above tests - complete blood count and chemistries - to proceed to surgery. This is often the case, and evaluation of each patient will allow the physician to eliminate unnecessary studies and diminish discomfort, cost, and delay for the patient.

However, there are many times when even the above studies will not be adequate to prepare a patient for surgery. This usually occurs in patients with multiple medical problems. The following special problems will be discussed: cardiac abnormalities, pulmonary dysfunction, diabetes mellitus, thyroid studies, and steroid preparation.

For a complete discussion of cardiac risks of surgery the reader is referred to the review articles by Goldman.[14,15] Briefly, his articles state that the cardiac risk can be estimated based on the severity of underlying heart failure, the occurrence of a recent myocardial infarction or various arrhythmias, the presence of aortic stenosis, and the patient's age and general medical condition. The three most important prognostic factors for increased cardiac risk are presence of an S_3 gallop or jugular venous distention on examination, a myocardial infarction within the past six months, and abnormal rhythms.[14,15]

Most of the methods in which cardiac risk can be reduced come under the aegis of the anaesthesiologist, such as maintaining adequate oxygenation and keeping the patient normotensive during the procedure. Cautious preoperative planning includes delaying surgery after a recent myocardial infarction, if possible; and treating any evidence of congestive failure with appropriate moderate diuresis.[14,15] In addition, although patients are usually kept NPO for at least eight hours before surgery, patients on cardiac medications should be allowed to take them with a small sip of water. This is especially true of beta-blockers and calcium-channel blockers.

Tisi has written an excellent review of preoperative evaluation of pulmonary function.[26] His article discusses pulmonary risk factors and prophylactic measures to avoid pulmonary dysfunction in the perioperative period. Tisi listed the following as candidates for evaluation of pulmonary function (by arterial blood gas and/or pulmonary function testing): patients with long, significant smoking histories; very elderly patients (over 70 years old); patients with a history of pulmonary problems such as chronic bronchitis or asthma; morbidly obese patients, and patients with severe scoliosis.[26] In addition, because of the risk of fat embolism after major trauma, a baseline arterial blood gas is indicated.

Tisi notes an increased incidence of pulmonary morbidity among patients with an arterial pCO_2 > 45 mm Hg, or on pulmonary function testing, those with a maximal breathing capacity less than 50% of predicted values, or an FEV_1 less than 2.0 liters. He also notes that arterial pO_2 by itself is not a reliable predictor of pulmonary morbidity.[26]

Finally Tisi mentions several prophylactic measures that should be performed to decrease pulmonary morbidity perioperatively. Preoperatively, patient education should include hyperinflation breathing techniques, cessation of smoking, and bronchodilation when indicated by results of pulmonary testing. Bronchodilation can be achieved by beginning treatment with nebulized metaproteranol and, if necessary, administration of an aminophylline drip on the night before surgery. Also, as with cardiac medications, all oral bronchodilators should be continued prior to surgery by giving them with a small sip of water.[26]

Postoperatively, the most important prophylactic measures are particular attention to hyperinflation, encouragement to cough, mobilization of secretions, control of pain, and early ambulation, if possible. Recommended standard orders are "TCDB q2 degrees" - turn, cough, and deep-breath, every 2 hours; and "blow-bottles to bedside for q1 degrees use." Blow-bottles are breathing tubes that encourage lung hyperinflation by having the patient attempt to raise three balls to the top of the bottle with a vigorous exhalation.[26]

The patient with diabetes mellitus is at increased risk for infection post-operatively. Controlling the serum glucose may decrease this risk, and this should be a major concern.[10,18,24] This is difficult perioperatively, however, because of a number of factors: 1) the patient is kept NPO the night before surgery; 2) he/she may not eat well for a day or two after surgery; 3) the stress of surgery will often trigger a hyperglycemic reaction; and 4) the patient will be immobilized postoperatively thereby decreasing the natural tendency for exercise to lower the serum glucose.

Preoperatively, the patient's insulin requirements are usually adjusted downward because of the decreased food intake. On the morning of surgery, all NPH insulin should be withheld because it will take effect much later in the day when the patient's glucose stores may be depleted. If the patient is on a low dose of regular insulin, it can simply be omitted. If the patient takes more than 10 units of regular insulin, it is usually halved and then given as regular insulin. In addition, patients on insulin should receive intravenous fluids containing some dextrose starting the night prior to surgery . A good compromise solution is D2.5W, as D5W will often significantly elevate serum glucose values. Patients taking an oral hypoglycemic agent should usually have it withheld on the morning of surgery.

If there is any doubt about the dosage of insulin to be given on the morning of surgery, a finger-stick glucose can be checked by one of several currently available methods. This gives an approximation of the serum glucose usually accurate to about 50 mg/dl. A sliding scale of regular insulin can then be ordered so that patients with an elevated glucose on the morning of surgery receive an appropriate amount of insulin. Patients on oral hypoglycemics can be managed in a similar manner.

Postoperatively, sliding-scale regular insulin is also the treatment commonly used to adjust insulin values for the various changing parameters of the postsurgical period. The glucose is assessed by finger-sticks at regular intervals. When the patient is not yet eating but only being fed intravenously, the interval should be every six hours. Once he is eating, the glucose is better monitored at each meal and at bedtime (ac and hs). Once the patient resumes eating a regular diet, his preoperative insulin regimen can be resumed but should be supplemented with a sliding scale of lesser magnitude.

One method of writing the sliding scale orders is as follows:

< 100	No units and call house officer (HO)
100-200	No units
200-300	x units
300-400	2x units
> 400	3x units and call HO

The "x" is determined by taking the patient's normal daily dosage of regular insulin and dividing it by the number of times he will receive insulin daily.

Patients with thyroid abnormalities who require medication should be kept on them during the preoperative period. As with cardiac and pulmonary medications, these can be given with a sip of water on the morning of surgery.

If it is necessary for a patient to take several medications prior to surgery, a significant amount of water may be ingested even when using small sips. Because of the potential problems with anaesthesia, these cases should be discussed preoperatively with the anaesthesiologist. It may be possible to substitute a parenteral drug for some of the medications.

Special consideration must be given to patients who are taking cortico-steroids or who have taken them within the past six months.[18,24] Because the oral steroid suppresses the patient's own immune system, the patient may be unable to mount the appropriate response to the stress of surgery. These patients should be supplemented with steroids preoperatively. A standard preoperative boost is as follows: cortisone acetate 100 mg IM at midnight and 6 a.m. the morning of surgery, and three or four postoperative doses given q8 hours.

Regional Anaesthesia

Many orthopaedic surgical procedures can be performed under local or regional anaesthesia thereby reducing time, expense, and the morbidity of general or spinal anaesthesia. In addition, fractures and dislocations require adequate anaesthesia both for the comfort of the patient and the doctor, who will find them much more easily reduced. Remember one rule all orthopaedists learn quickly: fractures hurt - a lot.

It is imperative to realize that the objective of any regional block is to inject the anaesthetic into the perineural tissue and not into the nerve. Direct injection of any substance into a nerve may injure the nerve.

The most commonly used anaesthetics for regional anaesthetic are lidocaine (Xylocaine), which has rapid onset (1-3 minutes) and is of short duration (1-2 hours); and bupivacaine (Marcaine, Sensorcaine), which is of slightly slower onset (2-10 minutes) and much longer duration (about 7-10 hours).

The most common complication from lidocaine is lowering the seizure threshold. The absolute maximum that should be given at any one time locally is 4.5 mg/kg if used without epinephrine, and 7 mg/kg if used with epinephrine. Bupivacaine also can lower the seizure threshold, but a more serious complication is cardiac arrhythmias which can occur if a large dose is injected intravenously. Bupivacaine is not approved for use in children. In normal sized adults, the maximum dose that should be given locally is 175 mg without epinephrine or 225 mg with epinephrine.

In all injections of local anaesthetic, it is mandatory to aspirate before injecting to avoid complications from intravenous injections.

Hematoma Block: Hematoma blocks are most commonly given prior to reduction of a Colles' fractures, but they can theoretically be given after almost any fracture. To perform a hematoma block, it is necessary to be able to palpate the fracture site. In fractures in which this cannot be done because of extreme swelling, usually old fractures, this technique must be abandoned.

Prior to giving the hematoma block, the area for injection should be sterilely prepared as thoroughly as for a surgical procedure. Failure to do this may introduce bacteria into the fracture site, effectively creating a contaminated, open fracture. After skin preparation, the fracture site is again palpated, using sterile gloves, and the needle is introduced into the fracture site, withdrawing on the syringe while entering. When the hematoma is entered, dark blood will return into the syringe. When this occurs, the local anaesthetic can be introduced into the fracture site. For Colles' fractures, 5 ml of lidocaine or bupivacaine are usually adequate. For tibial or ankle fractures, 10 ml are usually needed. It is wise to caution the patient beforehand that the injection, though used to anaesthetize the fracture site, is not without significant pain.

While the hematoma block is effective in relieving pain, it does not produce muscle relaxation, which may be necessary for fracture reduction.

Digital Block:[21] Digital blocks can be given either from a dorsal or palmar approach. However, the dorsal approach is recommended since the dorsal skin is less sensitive. In either case, after thorough skin preparation, a 25-gauge needle is introduced between the metacarpal heads on both sides of the digit to be blocked, in the region of the neurovascular bundles. A proximal injection site is chosen to prevent vascular compression and occlusion, which could occur from circumferential fluid in the digit. Two to three ml of local anaesthetic are usually adequate for a digital block. For dorsal injuries, it is often necessary to infiltrate over the dorsum of the MCPJ area to block some of the dorsal sensory innervation. Because of the vasoconstrictive properties of epinephrine, anaesthetic without epinephrine should always be used for digital blocks.

Median and Ulnar Nerve Blocks at Wrist:[21] The median nerve lies directly under the palmaris longus tendon, or in its absence, just ulnar to the flexor carpi radialis. A 25-gauge needle is inserted at the proximal wrist crease until paraesthesias are encountered and then 5 ml of local anaesthetic are injected.

The ulnar nerve lies between the flexor carpi ulnaris tendon and the ulnar artery at the wrist. The mnemonic is ANT - artery, nerve, tendon. A 25-gauge needle is inserted between the arterial pulse and the tendon at the proximal wrist crease until paraesthesias are encountered, the needle is slightly withdrawn until the paraesthesias cease, and 5 ml of local anaesthetic are injected.

Axillary Block:[21] The cords of the brachial plexus surround the third part of the axillary artery. Anaesthesia of the entire arm can be obtained by blocking the cords in this area. Because of the risk of injection into the axillary artery, this is a potentially dangerous procedure best reserved for experienced practitioners in the operating room. Caution should be used, as direct intravascular injection can cause seizures and cardiac arrhythmias.

The technique begins with the patient lying with the arm abducted to 90 degrees with the arm slightly externally rotated. The axilla should be shaved and meticulously prepped. There are several ways to obtain the desired block. The arterial puncture technique will be described.

After palpating the axillary pulse, a 3.8 cm, 22-gauge needle is introduced while withdrawing on the syringe. When arterial blood is aspirated, the needle is very slowly advanced until blood can no longer be aspirated. The needle should now be out of the artery, but if it was advanced carefully, it should be in the sheath which surrounds the cords of the brachial plexus. Forty to fifty ml of local anaesthetic are then introduced. Digital pressure to control hematoma over the artery must then be maintained for several minutes.

Ankle Blocks:[4] Ankle blocks are difficult to give because five nerves must be blocked: posterior tibial, deep peroneal, superficial peroneal, sural, and saphenous nerves.

The entire foot and ankle should be sterilely prepared. Begin with the posterior tibial nerve. Find it by palapating the posterior tibial artery and then introduce the needle just posterior to the artery and perpendicular to the medial malleolus. Inject 5-10 ml of the anaesthetic.

To identify the superficial peroneal nerve, invert and plantarflex the foot. The nerve and its larger branches can be seen under the skin by shining a light on the dorsum of the foot. Introduce the needle two fingerbreadths superior to the tip of the lateral malleolus and inject subcutaneously across the anterior margin of the fibula extending over the tibia. Use 3-5 ml of anaesthetic.

The deep peroneal nerve is found by palpating the space between the tibialis anterior and the extensor hallucis longus at the level of the malleoli.

Direct the needle into this space and perpendicular to bone. Withdraw the needle 3-5 mm from the bone and then inject 5-7 ml of solution.

The sural nerve is just posterior to the peroneal tendons behind the lateral malleolus. Direct the needle one centimeter posterior to the tendons at the level of the lateral malleolus and inject 3-5 ml of anaesthetic subcutaneously.

The saphenous nerve may be blocked by subcutaneous infiltration of 3-5 ml of local anaesthetic one fingerbreadth superior to the tip of the medial malleolus along the medial aspect of the tibia.

Antibiotics and Orthopaedic Infections

Antibiotics are used in orthopaedics either prophylactically before elective procedures, or therapeutically in the face of an established infection.[1]

When used, prophylactic antibiotics should follow three guidelines: 1) they should be short term; 2) they should be high dose; and 3) they should be broad range. The most commonly used prophylactic antibiotics are first-generation cephalosporins. The literature has shown the cephalosporins to provide a prophylactic effect in certain cases.[1] Use of a concurrent aminoglycoside with a cephalosporin has been studied, but adding the aminoglycoside has not usually shown a statistical difference over the use of the cephalosporin alone.

Prophylactic antibiotics are definitely indicated in orthopaedics whenever a foreign material is implanted into the body - e.g., total joint replacements, or internal fixation devices for fractures. In no other case have they definitely been shown to decrease the risk of postoperative infection.[1]

Many orthopaedists still use prophylactic antibiotics for other cases, however. Because of the morbidity of septic arthritis or osteomyelitis, both of which are much more difficult to eradicate than a soft tissue infection, antibiotics tend to be used whenever a joint cavity or the cortex of bone is violated.

The antibiotics should be given 30 minutes to one hour prior to surgery so that the circulating serum level is high when the skin incision is made. Many physicians continue the antibiotics up to 72 hours after surgery, but 24-48 hours are probably adequate. A guideline often used is that the antibiotic is continued until any drains are removed.

Antibiotics are commonly used by orthopaedists in the treatment of established bone and joint infections. However, the basic surgical principle of draining an established abscess must still be followed in orthopaedics. In cases of abscess formation, incision and drainage of the infection must precede antibiotic coverage to be effective.

Because of the difficulty of obtaining a culture from bones and joints, it is imperative to perform one culture to identify the infecting organism. Thus, antibiotics should <u>not</u> be given prior to the surgical procedure which is intended to drain an established infection and culture an abscess. If given before this procedure, the antibiotics may sterilize the culture and prevent the microbiology laboratory from being able to grow and identify the organism.

In cases where no definite abscess exists and a surgical procedure is not definitely planned, therapeutic antibiotics may be used expectantly. In these cases, it is helpful to know the most common infecting organisms.

In osteomyelitis (acute and chronic) and septic arthritis, the most common organism in most populations is *Staphylococcus aureus*. Among noncompromised hosts, this is true for all age groups with one exception. In young children between six months and two years, septic arthritis is more commonly caused by *Haemophilus influenzae*. The recommended drugs of choice and duration of use for many orthopaedic infections are listed below in Tables 9-1 and 9-2.

There are specific exceptions to the above rules. These include compromised hosts, specific traumatic inoculations, and total joint replacements. Table 9-1 lists many of these special cases and the most common infecting organisms in such instances.

TABLE 9-1

Orthopaedic Infections

Osteomyelitis	Newborn infant	*Staph. aureus*	PRSP + P Ceph 3
		Enterobacteriaceae	
		Group A, B strep	
	Child <= 3 yrs	*H. influenzae*	Cefuroxime or
		Streptococci	P Ceph 3
	Child > 3 yrs	*Staph. aureus*	PRSP
	Blood dyscrasia	*Staph. aureus*	PRSP +
		Salmonella sp.	P Ceph 3
		Enterobacteriaceae	
	Drug addicts	*Staph. aureus*	Ciprofloxacin
		Enterobacteriaceae	or ofloxacin
		Pseudomonas	
Foot Cellulitis	Diabetes m.	Polymicrobic	IMP or TC/CL
			or AM/BLI
	Penetrating wd.	*Pseudomonas*	P Ceph 3 AG or
			TC/CL or IMP
Hand Cellulitis	Dog/cat bite	*Pasteurella*	AM/CL
	Human bite	*Eikinella*	AM/CL
Muscle	"Gas gangrene"	*Cl. perfringens*	Hi-dose Pen G
			Wide debridement
			Hyperbaric O_2

Septic Arthritis	Infant < 3 mos.	*Staph. aureus*	PRSP + P Ceph 3
		Enterobacteriaceae	or APAG
		Group B strep	
	Child 3 mo-2 yrs	*H. influenzae*	PRSP +
		Pneumococci	cefuroxime
		Staph. aureus	
	Child > 2 yrs	*Staph. aureus*	PRSP +
		Group A strep	cefuroxime
		H. influenzae	
	Adult	*Gonococci* (>50%)	Imipenam
	Non-GC Adult	*Staph. aureus* (40%)	Imipenam
		Group A strep (27%)	
		Enterobacter. (23%)	
	? Venereal dz	*Gonococci*	Pen G or Ampicillin
	Joint prosthesis	*Staph. epi.* (40%)	Vancomycin +
		Staph. aureus (20%)	aztreonam
		Enterobacter.	
		Pseudomonas	
Septic Bursitis		*Staph. aureus*	PRSP
		M. tuberculosis	Consult for both
		M. marinum	Mycobacteria (rare)

AM/CL	=	Amoxicillin clavulanate
AM/BLI	=	Ampicillin/beta lactamase inhibitor
APAG	=	Antipseudomonal aminoglycoside
AP Pen	=	Anti-pseudomonal penicillins
IMP	=	Imipenem/cilastatin
P Ceph 3	=	Parenteral third-generation cephalosporins
P Ceph 3 AG	=	Parenteral third-generation cephalosporin with anti-pseudomonal activity
PRSP	=	Penicillinase resistant synthetic penicillin
TC/CL	=	Ticarcillin clavulanate

(Reprinted with permission from *Guide to Antimicrobial Therapy 1989*, Jay P. Sanford, M.D., author and publisher.)

[Refer to standard texts or Sanford's monograph for dosage guidelines.]

TABLE 9-2

Suggested Duration of Antibiotic Therapy

Site	Clinical Diagnosis	Duration (Days)
Bone	Acute osteomyelitis	42
	Chronic osteomyelitis	*
Joint	Septic arthritis	21
	Gonococcal arthritis (PCN R_x)	3
	Gonococcal arthritis (Other)	7
Skin	Cellulitis	**

* Until erythrocyte sedimentation rate normal (often more than three months).
** Until 3 days after acute inflammation disappears.

(Reprinted with permission from *Guide to Antimicrobial Therapy 1988*, Jay P. Sanford, M.D., author and publisher.)

Anticoagulation and Pulmonary Embolism[3,9, 17,19,23]

Venous thromboembolism is a common problem in orthopaedic surgery. Patients undergoing total hip replacement have a 30-50% risk of developing a deep venous thrombosis, with a 10% risk of pulmonary embolism and a mortality of 1-2% from either of these two factors.[19] Deep venous thrombi have been found in 70% of patients being operated on for hip fractures. One study showed total knee replacement to carry an 80% risk of deep venous thrombosis.[19]

Virchow established the three factors primarily responsible for the formation of vascular thrombosis: 1) stasis, 2) endothelial damage, and 3) a "hypercoagulable state."[23] Clinical risk factors that increase the risk of thromboembolism are advanced age, past history of thromboembolism, prolonged immobilization, malignant disease, obesity, varicose veins, oral contraceptive use, and congestive heart failure. The greatest risk factor is a past history of thromboembolism. These patients carry a four-fold greater risk of developing thromboembolic problems than the average elective surgical patient.[17]

Orthopaedic patients are at high risk for venous stasis because they are so often immobilized and unable to walk after surgery. Hull, in a recent review article, classified patients as low-, moderate- and high-risk and placed all orthopaedic patients having a major procedure on the lower limbs in the high-risk category.[17]

Deep venous thrombosis is painful and uncomfortable to the patient but, by itself, causes minimal morbidity. The danger is the possibility of a thrombus migrating to the lungs and causing a pulmonary embolism. Pulmonary embolism is the third most common cause of death in the United States and is a common cause of "sudden death." In fact, two-thirds of patients who die from a pulmonary embolism do so within 30 minutes after the acute event. This is often before they are seen by a nurse or physician. It has been estimated that the routine use of effective prophylactic measures in patients undergoing elective surgery could prevent 4,000-8,000 postoperative deaths each year in the United States.[23]

Because of the morbidity and mortality of treating an established pulmonary embolism, the treatment of choice in orthopaedics is to prevent the incidence of deep venous thrombosis by prophylactic anticoagulation in the perioperative period. Though that statement is easily defended, the problem becomes one of choosing a prophylactic agent.

The most thoroughly tested prophylactic measures are low-dose subcutaneous heparin, intravenous dextran, oral anticoagulants, and intermittent pneumatic compression of the legs. These have been studied both singly and in various combinations. A recent combination approach studied in orthopaedics has been the use of low-dose subcutaneous heparin with the oral venoconstrictor dihydroergotamine. These five measures will be considered separately. Among oral anticoagulants we will mention specifically warfarin sodium. Oral antiplatelet agents, such as aspirin and dipyridamole, have very limited use in the prevention of venous thromboembolism.

Many orthopaedic patients who develop a deep venous thrombosis do so **during the surgical procedure**. This problem has been estimated to occur in as many as 35% of patients undergoing major lower extremity surgery. It would then be prudent to begin any prophylaxis prior to the surgical procedure. Many regimens recommend it, but this does carry a higher risk of bleeding during surgery.

Low-Dose Subcutaneous Heparin: Low-dose heparin prevents thrombosis by inhibiting the coagulation cascade. It accelerates the rate of inhibition of the coagulation factors XII_a, XI_a, IX_a, X_a, and thrombin by antithrombin III.

A recommended regimen for the use of low-dose heparin is a dose of 5,000 units given two hours preoperatively, and then every twelve or eight hours postoperatively. This regimen has been termed "one of the measures of choice in preventing venous thromboembolism in moderate- and high-risk general surgical patients." Unfortunately, several studies have shown low-dose heparin to be less effective in hip surgery, and it is not considered the prophylaxis of choice in this group.

Low-dose heparin has the advantage that it does not require anticoagulant monitoring. The only associated significant clinical risk is the development of heparin-induced thrombocytopenia, but this has not been reported after its use in orthopaedic patients.

Intermittent Pneumatic Leg Compression: Intermittent pneumatic leg compression prevents venous thrombosis by enhancing blood flow in the deep veins of the legs and preventing venous stasis. In patients undergoing hip surgery, it has been shown to be effective in preventing calf-vein thrombosis. Unfortunately, compression of the calf has had minimal effect on thigh-vein thrombosis.

Recently, combined calf and thigh intermittent compression systems have been developed. It may be more effective in patients after hip surgery, but it may also be difficult to use in those patients because of pain around the incision site. It also cannot be used for knee, ankle, and foot surgery. Because of the difficulty in its use, it is not used frequently in orthopaedic surgery other than in spinal surgery. This is unfortunate because intermittent pneumatic leg compression is virtually free of clinically important side effects and can be used safely in patients who have a high risk of bleeding.

Oral Anticoagulants (Warfarin Sodium): Warfarin sodium prevents thrombosis by inhibiting the synthesis of the vitamin K-dependent coagulation factors (II, VII, IX, X). Multiple studies have shown it to be effective in preventing venous thrombosis and pulmonary embolism, and it is very effective in patients undergoing hip surgery.

Warfarin sodium does not take effect quickly, as it inhibits only the formation of new coagulation factors. Thus, its effectiveness only occurs after the circulating factors have been removed from the circulation. Clinically, this occurs 36-48 hours after the first dose of warfarin sodium is given. Because of the delayed effectiveness, the use of warfarin sodium almost mandates its use preoperatively as well as postoperatively.

Warfarin sodium prophylaxis carries with it a high risk of clinically significant bleeding problems. Its use must be monitored daily by the prothrombin time ratio during the induction of prophylaxis, and then at least weekly after a steady state is reached. The normal prothrombin ratio is 1.0. The amount the ratio should be increased varies according to the reagent the laboratory is using to measure the value. One should check with the hospital's clinical laboratory and/or a hematologist to determine the ratio which provides a safe, yet clinically significant anticoagulant effect.

Because of the need to administer warfarin sodium preoperatively, and the associated high risk of bleeding problems, its routine clinical use is questionable. One recent study recommended beginning warfarin sodium 10-14 days preoperatively in very low doses, and then increasing the dose immediately after surgery. This achieved a clinically significant decrease in venous thrombosis with no increase in operative and postoperative bleeding complications.

Dextran: Dextran is a glucose polymer that works as a volume expander. Its anticoagulation effect has been attributed to decreased blood viscosity, reduced platelet interaction with damaged vessel walls, and an increased tendency for fibrin clots to undergo fibrinolysis. Dextran is a heparinoid with similar effects to heparin but is much less potent.

Dextran polymer is clinically available in two sizes: dextran 70 with a mean molecular weight of 70,000 and dextran 40 with a mean molecular weight of 40,000. Dextran 40 is the size used most often for prophylaxis. It has been shown to be an effective prophylaxis in moderate-risk and high-risk surgical patients (including hip surgery). The regimens have varied but most include starting the dextran at the time of surgery and continuing it for several days postoperatively in a dose of 50 ml/hour for between 4-6 hours daily.

Dextran is tolerated well by most patients but may cause volume overload problems in patients with cardiac dysfunction or the elderly with unrecognized cardiac impairment. It can cause occasional hypersensitivity reactions and also can cause headaches and nausea.

Low-Dose Subcutaneous Heparin with Dihydroergotamine: As mentioned above, low-dose subcutaneous heparin has been called a "measure of choice" for preventing venous thrombosis in moderate- and high-risk surgical patients, but it has less effectiveness in patients undergoing hip surgery. Dihydroergotamine mesylate is a vasoconstrictor that acts on the veins (capacitance vessels) while having little effect on the arterioles (resistance vessels). By causing constriction of venous smooth muscle, it increases venous tone and decreases venous stasis.

A recent prospective multi-center study showed that low-dose heparin combined with oral dihydroergotamine mesylate (DHE) was effective in preventing deep venous thrombosis in patients undergoing total hip replacement.[3] This study confirmed the results of other similar studies. The study compared the heparin/DHE group to a placebo group and found no significant difference between the two groups in the rate of hemorrhagic complications or other adverse reactions.

In this study the regimen was 5,000 units of heparin with 0.5 mg of DHE given subcutaneously two hours preoperatively and then every eight hours for 7-9 days postoperatively.

The most significant concern about DHE is its potential to cause vasospasm with the attendant problems with coronary or cerebral vasospasm. Earlier studies showed an annual incidence of vasospasm of 0.01% with the use of DHE but this incidence has dropped to 0.003% since 1983, apparently because of stricter adherence to recommended dosage guidelines.[3]

In summary, no ideal method of prophylaxis against deep venous thrombosis exists. However, because of the frequency and severity of the problem, some form of prophylaxis is indicated. While subcutaneous heparin is adequate for many orthopaedic procedures, its use in hip surgery has not been shown to be effective, and it should either be supplemented with dihydroergotamine or another form of prophylaxis should be used, such as warfarin sodium or dextran.

Fat Embolism Syndrome[11,12]

Fat embolism is an important cause of acute respiratory distress syndrome (ARDS) that often occurs after major trauma. The incidence has been estimated as occurring in 10-15% of patients with long bone fractures, and possibly higher in patients with multiple fractures or pelvic fractures. It is a serious complication as mortality rates related to fat embolism have been reported between 5 and 15%.

Fat embolism is a clinical diagnosis that classically manifests itself approximately 72 hours after major trauma. However, it may occur earlier and signs and symptoms of the syndrome are evident in 60% of patients within 24 hours after major trauma and in 85% of patients within 48 hours.

Tachycardia and tachypnea are the first clinical signs of fat embolism syndrome. Tachypnea is often followed by dyspnea which may be accompanied by cyanosis. Shortly after this occurs, confusion and other changes in mental status may occur if the syndrome worsens. Petechiae develop in about 50% of patients with fat embolism. The petechiae have a well-demarcated distribution, usually occurring across the root of the neck, axilla, and especially in the conjunctivae. Retinal lesions can also be identified on funduscopic examination.

Respiratory failure is the major pathophysiologic abnormality in the fat embolism syndrome. It manifests itself as arterial hypoxemia and serial arterial blood gas measurements are a necessity if the syndrome is suspected. The critical laboratory finding is a low PaO_2. Serial chest roentgenograms will occasionally reveal fluffy exudates in the lung fields. A ventilation-perfusion scan of the lungs will reveal small, but widespread embolic phenomena within the lung fields.

Treatment of the fat embolism syndrome requires a high index of suspicion to identify it early and prevent the onset of severe respiratory failure. Treatment is mainly aimed at respiratory support by administration of oxygen and ventilatory assistance by endotracheal intubation, if necessary. Other treatment options used include the administration of steroids, intravenous alcohol, low-dose heparin, or low molecular weight dextran. Currently, none of these is thought to change the prognosis, and current recommended treatment is merely respiratory support as soon as the syndrome is suspected.

Extremity Neurovascular Status[7,20]

Many orthopaedic procedures and fractures place the injured extremity at risk for neurovascular compromise. The results of an ignored neurovascular injury can be catastrophic. These include Volkmann's ischemic contracture of the upper extremity and the compartment syndromes. In the postoperative or postreduction period, the neurovascular system must be carefully monitored. *On noting any change in the neurovascular status of the extremity, intervention must be aggressive and prompt.*

In many injuries, it is not necessary to admit the patient to the hospital for monitoring. A responsible adult can be instructed in the signs and symptoms of neurovascular compromise and told to return to the emergency department should they develop. Some musculoskeletal injuries are at high risk for compromise, and these patients should be admitted for strict elevation and monitoring (e.g., displaced pediatric supracondylar fractures, tibial shaft fractures, knee dislocations).

The examiner must serially monitor several parameters of the patient's injured extremity. These include peripheral pulses, sensation, temperature, capillary refill, and motor function. Always look for any of the four "P's" which may suggest a compartment syndrome (pain, pallor, paresthesias, and pulselessness).

Peripheral Pulses: When possible, the peripheral pulses should be monitored distal to the injury. Often circular casts will prevent accesss to the pulses; however, soft, bulky dressings can be split to provide limited access to the peripheral pulse distal to the injury or surgical procedure. The measurement should be compared with the contralateral side when possible. The presence of a pulse does not eliminate the possibility of a compartment syndrome. In the older patient population, Doppler evaluation may be necessary to detect flow in the distal pulses.

In extremities that are at significant risk for arterial compromise, such as knee dislocations, the physician may wish to obtain an arteriogram of the extremity to ensure the integrity of the arterial system. In injuries such as a knee dislocation, patients are at risk for late occlusion of the arterial system caused by an intimal flap. Many orthopaedists recommend that all knee dislocations recieve an arteriogram, as the rate of arterial injury is significant. Absence of a pulse in a patient with a knee dislocation is a surgical emergency. Delay in awaiting an arteriogram may result in loss of limb. The arteriogram should be obtained in the operating room or else omitted in favor of immediate exploration of the popliteal artery.

Sensibility: Sensibility should be carefully tested over the entire extremity involved in the injury. The initial evaluation and recording of this information is critical, as it forms the basis for comparison for subsequent examinations. The upper extremity sensibility examination should include evaluating the autogenous zones of the medial, ulnar, and radial nerves. Two-point discrimination, as described by Moberg, is a rapid, accurate and reproducible assessment of digital sensation. In the lower extremity, the testing should include the autonomous areas of the dermatomes. The patient should be questioned about the development of paresthesias in the injured extremity.

The sensory exam can be misleading in the perioperative period when a tourniquet has been used on the extremity. Long periods of tourniquet ischemia will often give transient paresthesias and occasional numbness. The sensory deficit caused by the tourniquet will usually improve with time. If it does not, the examiner should realize that continued deterioration in the postoperative exam may be a sign of a compartment syndrome.

Temperature: An assessment of the temperature of the injured extremity should be included in the examination. In most cases, temperature is checked by comparing the injured extremity to the uninjured extremity. A beneficial aid following replantation or revascularization of a severely injured extremity is a temperature monitor placed on the distal extremity. A rapid fall in the temperature of a replanted digit often is the first sign of impending vascular compromise. When the sympathetic nervous system remains intact to the injured extremity, the temperature probes are less reliable.

Capillary Refill: Capillary refill, pulp turgor, and the appearance of the digits give information about both the arterial and venous circulation. The color of the pulp of the digits gives information regarding venous outflow. If the pulp of the digit is engorged and purple, venous drainage is sluggish. When the pulp has pallor, the arterial circulation may be diminished. The amount of time necessary for the pulp to blush after blanching with pressure is known as the capillary refill. Subjective terms are used to describe the capillary refill time - good, fair, or sluggish. Capillary refill can be more accurately described, however, in the amount of time it takes for the pulp of the digit to recover its normal color. Normally, this takes less than two seconds. A slow capillary refill is a sign of vascular compromise. The capillary refill should always be compared with the contralateral side. The most reliable area to check for capillary refill is midway between the pulp of the digit and the lateral border of the nailplate.

Motor Function: Motor function of the extremity is included in the neurovascular assessment. Specific neuromuscular units can be evaluated despite dressings or casts. In the upper extremity, a motor unit innervated by each of the three major motor nerves to the forearm and hand should be examined. This can be done quickly by asking the patient to "hitchhike your thumb" (EPL - radial nerve), "cross your fingers" (finger intrinsics - ulnar nerve), and "touch the tips of your fingers with your thumb" (opposition - median nerve).

For lower extremity injuries, the leg is often placed in plaster. For evaluation, the patient is asked to dorsiflex and plantarflex the toes. Dorsiflexion of the great toe is especially important to check as this tests the EHL and the deep peroneal nerve, which is commonly injured. Be certain the patient actually dorsiflexes the toe, rather than simply passively rebounding from plantar flexion. This can often be mistaken for active function of the EHL. Passive motion testing is also important, as pain associated with the passive motion is the hallmark for compartment syndrome. An unreliable assessment is to ask the patient to "wiggle your toes" as he or she may flex toes and simply allow them to rebound to the neutral position - which is not a true test of toe extension.

Treatment of Neurovascular Compromise: The etiology of neurovascular compromise can be separated into extrinsic and intrinsic causes. Extrinsic causes include tight dressings, splints, or casts. All constriction should be removed immediately upon the suspicion of compromise. If a cast has been previously split, it should be resplit to the the skin. Dried blood in the cast padding can cause a constriction similar to a cast. All dressings should also be split to expose the skin. In some hand injuries, especially replantations, the removal of a few sutures may relieve the constriction caused by postoperative edema in the replanted part.

After the dressings have been split and the wound inspected, intrinsic causes of neurovascular compromise must be considered. The differential diagnosis includes compartment syndrome, vasospasm (secondary to cold, pain, or anxiety), late presentation of an arterial injury, or impending failure of a replanted digit or free tissue transfer secondary to vascular occlusion.

Types of Immobilization

In the perioperative period most orthopaedic patients are immobilized in some manner. The degree of immobilization varies, depending upon the extent of the procedure and the security of the internal fixation, if any.

Soft Dressings: These dressings consist of a combination of gauze, sheet cotton, or Webril and compression bandages. The dressings serve to cover the wounds, and give compression over the operative site. A useful dressing in knee injuries is to apply several layers of sheet cotton from midcalf to midthigh. The area is then wrapped with bias stockinette, or elastic bandages for additional compression. This bulky dressing is called a Jones' dressing and has been shown to decrease edema with minimal risk of extrinsic compression.[5]

There are several commercially available immobilization aids that are extremely useful. These include knee immobilizers, shoulder immobilizers and arm slings. The knee immobilizer is an alternative to casting and maintains the knee in an extended postion. It can be removed for bathing or physical therapy. A major disadvantage to the knee immobilizer is the fit is not always accurate, and the immobilizer often slides below the knee. In addition, the knee immobilizer offers little compression. In order to add compression to the knee immobilizer, and improve fit, a Jones' dressing can be placed on the knee prior to application of the knee immobilizer.

The shoulder immobilizer is useful in immobilizing the shoulder postoperatively, and after the reduction of a shoulder dislocation. Additional padding should be placed beneath the wrist, at the elbow, and in the axilla for comfort. Slings serve little purpose in the perioperative period, as they place the extremity in the dependent position.

Dressings with Plaster Splints: In order to achieve immobilization, compression, and additional protection, plaster splints are often incorporated into postoperative dressings. This type of dressing is commonly used in hand injuries where a dorsal plaster slab is incorporated into the bulky hand dressing. The slab is extended onto the forearm for comfort and wrist stabilization. Frequently, it is advisable to incorporate the elbow in the splint for more reliable stabilization and to prevent migration of the splint. The application of splints on both the volar and dorsal aspects of the hand and forearm is rarely indicated except for stabilization of fractures about the hand or wrist.

The use of splints avoids the complications of circumferential casts. All types of splints described earlier can be utilized in the perioperative period. In the lower extremity, the posterior splint is commonly used as a dressing. In patients who require immobilization above the knee, it is often better to apply a long-leg cast, and bivalve it (splitting the cast on both the medial and lateral sides) in the recovery room.

Casts: Casts are routinely used in the perioperative period. There is some controversy over the necessity to split casts immediately after their application. Circumferential dressings predispose the patient to neurovascular compromise; however, the cast maintains better alignment than a splint. A general recommendation about splitting casts is to split the cast whenever there is doubt about the development of neurovascular compromise. In the unresponsive patient, casts should be avoided as a postoperative dressing. The patient would be better managed with splints, and changed to a definitive cast after resolution of perioperative edema. Any loss of position caused by splitting a cast can be recovered after the acute edema of surgery has resolved.

Details about placing the various types of casts can be found in Chapter Seven (*Casting and Splinting Techniques*).

Traction: Traction has limited use in the perioperative period. It is used to immobilize open fractures in patients undergoing multiple debridements prior to a definitive procedure. Traction is also a useful method to obtain elevation of the extremity. Details about setting up the various types of traction can be found in Chapter Eight (*Traction Techniques*).

Prosthetics and Orthotics

It is beyond the scope of this manual to give a complete discussion of the many orthoses and prostheses available on the market. An extremity prosthesis is a very useful tool after a congenital or traumatic amputation. The major limitation of the upper extremity prosthesis is the lack of sensibility at the terminal device. This lack of sensibility limits the amount of fine motor function possible. In the lower extremity, normal gait was limited in the past by a lack of push-off. This lack of push-off has recently been improved with the development of energy storing devices.

Prosthetics

Upper Extremity Prosthetics:[2] There are several types of upper extremity prostheses on the market today that vary with the level of the amputation. The two most common types are the myoelectric and mechanical. In the normal extremity, the elbow and shoulder function to position the sensate hand in space. To operate a conventional above-elbow prosthesis, the amputee must use the scapulothoracic joint, and opposite shoulder to power both the terminal device and perform elbow flexion and extension. This is performed by operating a series of switches to first position the terminal device in space, and then activate the terminal device. This is cumbersome for most wearers, and the device is often used by the unilateral amputee as a cosmetic replacement, and helper hand. Many unilateral above-elbow amputees choose not to use a prosthesis because they are so difficult to operate. However, patients with bilateral amputations will often become quite adept at the use of above-elbow prostheses as they must rely on them for all activities of daily living.

Below-elbow amputees often become good prosthetic users. The terminal device is also activated by a shoulder harness using scapulothoracic motion. Having an intact shoulder and elbow joint allows the user to easily position the terminal device in space. There are several terminal devices available to the amputee, including voluntary opening, and voluntary closing hooks and hands. The terminal device is usually chosen by the wearer, depending on his job requirements and extent of use of the prosthesis.

In the myoelectric arm, the user triggers electrodes inside the socket to open and close the terminal device. With some practice, the user can become very adept at manipulating the prosthesis. This prosthesis is cosmetically acceptable as it resembles the normal hand, and it is gaining popularity among the younger prosthetic users. A significant drawback to the myoelectric prosthesis is the high initial cost, and a higher maintenance cost. It is also slightly heavier.

Lower Extremity Prosthetics: There have been many recent advances in the engineering of the lower extremity prosthesis. The majority of the development surrounds the concept of storing energy in the prosthesis to allow for more normal push-off. One approach to this problem has been to incorporate carbon fibers into the foot of the prosthesis. These fibers are aligned much like the plantar aponeurosis, and give some spring at toe-off. This prosthesis is currently marketed under the tradename Carbon Copy II. An extension of the energy-storing concept has been to construct the entire foot and pylon of the prosthesis out of carbon fiber, taking into account the patient's weight, height, and length of stump. This prosthesis allows more energy storage, and the patient has the capacity to spring from the floor. The "energy storage" mechanism self-adjusts to the patients cadence, and an almost normal gait can be maintained even while running. This prosthesis is marketed under the trade name of Flex Foot.

The suspension systems for below-knee prostheses vary. In rare instances, the prosthesis is endbearing, but for most patients, some of the load is borne by the patellar tendon, i.e., patellar-tendon bearing (PTB). The prosthesis can be held on by extending it above the condyles of the femur, a supracondylar strap can be added, the prosthesis can be connected to a belt suspension system, or various forms of suction can be utilized.

The above-knee prosthesis incorporates a hinge at the knee to allow for a normal gait patttern. The hinge may be of one of several designs, free, friction, safety, and hydraulic. In all designs, the axis of the hinge is placed behind the mechanical axis of the prosthesis to allow the knee to be locked with hip extension. The simplest hinge at the knee joint, the free hinge, allows free articulation of the prosthesis. The drawback to this hinge is that the swing speed of the lower portion of the component is not controlled. The hydraulic knee, however, varies the length of the prosthetic swing phase to allow the gait to appear more normal. The disadvantage of the hydraulic knee is its initial expense, greater weight, and higher maintenance cost when compared with the single-axis free hinge. It is usually chosen by younger, more active individuals, often after traumatic amputations.

The hip disarticulation prosthesis adds a hinge at the level of the pelvis. With this prosthesis, a normal appearing gait is not possible. The wearer must power the prosthesis by tilting the pelvis. This gives the patient a lurch in the gait.

Orthotics

Upper Extremity Orthotics:[13] Upper extremity orthoses most often center around the wrist and hand. Orthotic splinting can be used for several purposes which include protection, maintainence of gains in ROM, to help mobilize contracted joints, and to stretch skin and scar. Splints can be applied to the hand in several modes: static, serial-static, and dynamic.

In diseases such as rheumatoid arthritis and cerebral palsy, static splints are used to maintain the hand in a functional postion. These splints are usually worn only at night. The splints consist of volar forearm and wrist segments fabricated from plastic to hold the wrist in a functional position, wrist dorsiflexed, metacarpophalangeal joints flexed to 90 degrees, proximal interphalangeal joints flexed to 10-20 degrees, and the distal interphalangeal joints extended.

Serial static splinting uses a number of static splints to gradually bring a deformity into the corrected postion. The splints are serially exchanged as range of motion increases after physical therapy. The splints are similar in design to the static splints, although the position of the hand is changed to conform to the deformity.

After trauma to the hand, orthoses are employed to maintain functional position. Rubber band outriggers are added to the serial splint to create passive range of motion. Early range of motion is important to the successful outcome of tendon repairs, especially flexor tendons. In the posttrauma patient, it is not uncommon for the patient to wear a dynamic splint during the day, and to protect the extremity with a static splint while sleeping.

Lower Extremity Orthotics:[22] There are a number of orthoses commercially available for the treatment of lower extremity pain. Many are used to treat foot pain of various etiologies. This discussion centers on some of the more common lower extremity injuries and their orthotic treatment.

Aids to the Longitudinal Arch: Many patients will develop planovalgus deformities of the foot (flatfeet). In many, this is not painful, and therefore requires no treatment. Should the condition become painful, a number of devices can be used to support the arch of the foot. These include felt medial arch supports, nonrigid molded shoe inserts, and molded rigid shoe inserts. All of these designs elevate the medial longitudinal arch of the foot, and reduce the subluxated talonavicular joint. In addition, the rigid orthosis can be molded to capture the calcaneus and act as an additional heel counter. The disadvantage of the rigid design is in the rigidity of the device not absorbing shock, and the cost of the custom-molded type.

Aids to Heel Position: The active athlete will occasionally present with shin splints. These are most often caused by valgus position of the heel, and over pronation of the feet. This is most successfully treated by a period of rest and the addition of a medial heel wedge to the inside of the shoe. Iliotibial band syndrome is another overuse syndrome and it is most often seen in patients with relative genu varum (bowlegs). One possible treatment for this is a lateral heel wedge in the shoe to help unload the lateral compartment of the knee.

Finally, plantar fasciitis is an inflamation of the insertion of the plantar aponeurosis to the calcaneus. This can be an overuse syndrome, and is most often seen after a rapid increase in activity. Treatment includes the use of medial arch support and heel cup or medial heel wedge.

Corrective Shoes: In some cases of metatarsus adductus in children, corrective shoes can be helpful in reducing the deformity. These shoes are reverse last, and the medial aspect of the shoe tends to put pressure on the metatarsals and direct them laterally. After correction has been obtained, recurrence of the deformity can be maintained with straight last shoes.

Often the treatment of metatarsus adductus was associated with the treatment of internal tibial torsion. In the past, nonoperative treatment of tibial torsion consisted of connecting shoes with a metal bar (Denis-Browne splint). This is no longer routinely recommended in the treatment of internal tibial torsion, as it will correct with growth in all but the most severe cases.

Ankle Orthoses: Most orthoses for the ankle have two purposes: to maintain foot position, and to aid in dorsiflexion of the foot. The best indication for the latter is a patient with a peroneal nerve palsy. The patient lacks active dorsiflexion, and has some medial-lateral instability. The orthosis can consist of metal uprights placed outside the shoe which have a hinge at the ankle and attach to a leather cuff on the calf, or can be a custom-molded plastic shell which fits the inside of the shoe. Both braces can be fabricated with varying amounts of plantar- and dorsiflexion to aid in gait. If hindfoot stability is a problem, the plastic AFO (ankle-foot orthosis) can be molded in the corrected position. In a metal orthosis, straps can be added to give additional hindfoot stability.

Knee Orthoses: Knee orthotics are used in the cruciate deficient knee to prevent translation of the tibia on the femur during sports activities. These braces are usually custom-fit to the patient and provide rigid three-point fixation. Much of the support of the brace comes from its limitation of terminal extension. More recently, off-the-shelf derotation braces have become available. The disadvantage of the custom fit brace is the high cost.

Additional orthotics for the knee are commonly used which provide little structural support to the knee. For example, a neoprene sleeve gives a sensation of support and maintains heat within the joint. Many athletes use a prophylactic hinged knee brace in attempts to prevent injury to the knee. This is an unsolved issue, as recent studies have shown no positive effect of the prophylatic knee brace in the prevention of knee injuries among college football players.[25]

The knee-ankle-foot orthosis (KAFO) is used in patients who have insufficient quadriceps strength to maintain the knee in full extension during gait. This orthosis is fabricated from molded polypropylene or double upright braces with leather cuffs. This brace allows for the knee to be locked into extension so the patient may walk with a straight-leg circumduction gait. Hinges are usually incorporated to allow the patient to sit comfortably.

Hip Orthoses: Bracing at the hip is difficult, as the joint is subject to the large stresses of the long lever arm of the leg. Most braces at the hip are fabricated to control rotation of the extremity at the hip. This is achieved by adding a pelvic band to the KAFO brace for better control of rotation.

A special brace that has been developed for the treatment of Legg-Calvé-Perthes disease is the abduction orthosis. This orthosis maintains the hips abducted and internally rotated, and thus places the femoral head deep into the acetabulum. The goal of the conservative treatment of Perthes disease is to contain the femoral head in the acetabulum while revascularization takes place. Many orthoses have been designed, the most common of which is the Scottish-Rite abduction orthosis. The merits of this orthosis are controversial, as it does not internally rotate the hip.

Another special orthosis used at the hip is a thigh lacer which is connected to a pelvic band. This brace prevents adduction, and maintains the hip reduced after total hip arthroplasty.

Spinal Orthoses: Orthotics for the spine can be categorized into two classes, corrective or stabilizing. The stabilizing orthotics include the corsets and molded polypropylene jackets which support the spine and attempt to maintain lordosis. These are used in postoperative and postinjury periods to support the spine, and limit the amount of bending allowed to the patient.

Corrective braces are used for the conservative treatment of scoliosis. These braces apply pressure to the spine at prescribed points in an attempt to straighten and derotate the curve. The timing and usefulness of bracing in scoliosis is a current debate. The Milwaukee brace consists of a molded girdle and steel superstructure which comes over the shoulders to the occiput and chin. Several corrective pads and irritators are attached to the brace to straighten the curve. The low-profile brace is an adaptation of the scoliosis brace which can be used for curves with the apex at or below T_8. This brace consists of molded polypropylene with corrective pads and irritators built inside the mold.

Physical Therapy

Preoperative and postoperative physical therapy plays a major role in the outcome of orthopaedic procedures. Many a technical operative success becomes a functional failure because the patient does not recover range of motion or motor strength. In addition, physical and occupational therapists play an integral role in the evaluation of patients with motor deficits, muscular dystrophy, or neural injury through careful manual motor testing and gait evaluations.

This discussion will not distinguish between the roles of the occupational therapist and the physical therapist. In general, the physical therapist deals with therapy aimed at motor strength and locomotion, while the occupational therapist is involved with hand therapy, and use of the extremities for activities of daily living. The borderline between the occupational therapist and the physical therapist is not well defined, and there is significant crossover.

Consideration of physical therapy needs should be evaluated preoperatively in the elective surgical patient. Preoperative physical therapy may assist in improving the patient's motor strength preoperatively, thus shortening the postoperative rehabilitation phase. The patient should be informed of the limitations of physical activity during the postoperative period. How long will the patient be wheelchair-bound or bedridden? What appliances will the patient need in order to ambulate? Can the patient reliably manage the weightbearing status prescribed by the surgeon? Will the patient require a brief rehabilitative stay in a skilled nursing facility?

In the trauma patient, physical therapy should begin as soon as the patient is stable from his injuries. Initial goals should be to maintain as much range of motion and muscle tone as possible. If injuries to the extremities have been stabilized, careful range of motion should be started. Early physical therapy is especially useful in preserving the range of motion and preventing contractures in the patient with a closed head injury. Inhibitory splints and casts can be used to prevent equinus deformities of the lower extremities. In addition, functional hand splints can be applied to prevent flexion contracture of the wrist. As these patients recover from their injuries, the therapy can be expanded to include active ROM and ambulation.

Protocols for physical therapy vary widely from institution to institution and from surgeon to surgeon. The following discussion offers several protocols for some common orthopaedic procedures. Weightbearing status after fracture fixation should be determined by the operating surgeon based on his assessment of the adequacy of reduction and stability of the fixation.

Rehabilitation After Anterior Cruciate Ligament Reconstruction

The rehabilitation of the knee after anterior cruciate ligament (ACL) reconstruction is a topic for much discussion. This rehabilitation protocol is currently used for ACL reconstructions using the iliotibial band and the semitendinosus in an over-the-top technique similar to the technique of Zarins.[27] It is also suitable for use after the technique of using a portion of patellar ligament with bone blocks at each end.

After reconstruction, wounds are closed over suction drains. The leg is placed in a hinged brace with 30-60 degrees of motion permitted. The brace is fitted preoperatively to allow accurate setting of the hinges. The drains are usually removed at 24-48 hours postsurgery, and the patient is permitted to begin ambulation, nonweightbearing on the operative side. Sutures are removed at 10 days, and the patient begins passive extension exercises of the knee, and active isometric hamstring strengthening. Continuous passive motion is utilized during this period if it is available. The current trend is towards allowing earlier passive extension of the knee, in some cases, immediately postoperatively.

Six weeks postoperatively, the patient is permitted to weightbear as tolerated out of brace and is weaned from crutches. Weaning from crutches is not possible until the patient has less than 10 degrees of flexion contracture of the knee. At this point, the patient is permitted to begin active range of motion of the hamstrings. Stationary bicycle and swimming are begun at 6 weeks.

At three months postoperatively, the patient is permitted to jog, and begin resistive quadriceps exercise. The patient is permitted to return to full competition in approximately nine months if comparison CYBEX testing demonstrates adequate hamstring and quadriceps strength.

Rehabilitation After Total Hip Arthroplasty

Currently, two types of implants are in use, cement fixation and biologic fixation. The patients who recieve biologic fixation implants generally have longer periods of protective touchdown weightbearing ambulation. There is a considerable benefit to the early mobilization of these patients in the prevention of postoperative pneumonia, maintenance of muscle tone, and prevention of pulmonary embolus.

After arthroplasty, the patient remains at bedrest on the day of surgery. While in bed, the patient often uses a triangular abduction pillow to prevent adduction and possible dislocation. On the first postoperative day, the patient is allowed out of bed to a chair with assistance. Careful attention must be paid to the patient's hematocrit, as it tends to drift downward after surgery, and the patient may require transfusion.

After removal of suction drains, at 24-48 hours postsurgery, the patient begins standing with touchdown weightbearing (TDWB) on the operative side using a walker or crutches. In cemented hips, some patients can be permitted to partial weightbear. In addition to ambulation, the patient learns transfers, and quadriceps, hamstring, and hip abduction exercises. The limited weightbearing status is maintained in the cemented prostheses for 4-6 weeks, while restricted weightbearing is usually maintained on the biologic fixation components for 3 months or longer.[8]

Rehabilitation After Hip Fracture

The rationale for the internal fixation of intertrochanteric and femoral neck fractures is for immediate mobilization of the patient postoperatively. In the patient in which a compression screw and side-plate have been used, ambulation will cause compression across the fracture site. The surgeon must be satisfied with the stability of the fracture before unrestricted ambulation is permitted. Usually, these patients are started on protective touchdown weightbearing with crutches or a walker.

In patients where an endoprosthesis is employed, the patient may be permitted immediate partial or even full weightbearing status as tolerated.

Rehabilitation After Total Knee Arthroplasty

Similar to total hip arthroplasty management, rehabilitation after total knee arthroplasty is dependent on whether the fixation used at surgery is cement or a porous-coated biological fixation method. The biological method requires bony ingrowth into the pores of the prosthesis and requires several months for fully stable fixation, thus requiring longer periods of restricted weightbearing.

After arthroplasty, the patient usually remains at bedrest on the day of surgery. On the first postoperative day, the patient is allowed out of bed to a chair with assistance. After removal of suction drains, at 24-48 hours postsurgery, the patient begins standing with touch down weightbearing (TDWB) on the operative side using a walker or crutches. With cemented knee implants, some patients can be permitted immediate partial weightbearing. In addition to ambulation, the patient learns transfers, and quadriceps, and hamstring exercises. In total knee arthroplasty, a most important consideration is regaining a range of motion after surgery. To this end, many surgeons require their patients to demonstrate 90 degrees flexion of the operated knee prior to discharge from the hospital. The limited weightbearing status is maintained in the cemented prostheses for 4-6 weeks, while restricted weightbearing is maintained on the biologic fixation components up to three months.

Rehabilitation of the Shoulder

The shoulder joint has the largest range of motion of any joint in the body. After arthroplasty or hemiarthroplasty the rehabilitation efforts can be classified into three phases. The first phase is passive or assisted motion of the shoulder. The second phase consists of active exercises, and the third phase consists of resistive muscle exercises. The goal of the rehabilitation program is to gain as much range of motion as possible, and to restore motor power. The progression of the patient through the rehabilitation program is dependent on the indications for the patient's surgery, most specifically, the integrity of the deltoid and rotator cuff musculature. If the rotator cuff was preserved during surgery, Hughes and Neer recommend isometric exercise as early as the 17th postoperative day.[16]

References

1. Antimicrobial prophylaxis in surgery. In: **The Medical Letter,** 29(750): 91-94, 09 October 1987.
2. Atkins DJ, Meier RH. *Comprehensive management of the upper limb amputee.* New York: Springer-Verlag, 1989.
3. Beisaw NE et al. Dihydroergotamine/heparin in the prevention of deep-vein thrombosis after total hip replacement. A controlled, prospective, randomized multicenter trial. **JBJS-A,** 70A(1): 2-10, 1988.
4. Beskin JL, Baxter DE. Regional anesthesia for ambulatory foot and ankle surgery. **Orthopaedics.** 10(1): 109-111, 1987.
5. Charnley J. *The Closed Treatment of Common Fractures.* Edinburgh: Churchill-Livingstone, 1972.
6. Collins JA. Blood transfusions and disorders of surgical bleeding. In: Sabiston DC Jr, ed. *Textbook of Surgery: The Biological Basis of Modern Surgical Practice.* 13th edition. Philadelphia: W. B. Saunders, 1986.
7. Connolly JF. *Fracture Complications: Recognition, Prevention, Management.* Chicago: Yearbook Medical Publishers, 1988.
8. Crenshaw AH, ed. *Campbell's Operative Orthopaedics.* 7th edition. St. Louis: C. V. Mosby, 1987.
9. Dalen JE et al. Venous thromboembolism: scope of the problem. **Chest,** 89(5) [Supplement]: 370S-373S, 1986.
10. Davis JH. Surgical aspects of diabetes mellitus. In: Sabiston DC Jr, ed. *Textbook of Surgery: The Biological Basis of Modern Surgical Practice.* 13th edition. Philadelphia: W. B. Saunders, 1986: 151-157.
11. Evarts CMcC. The fat embolism syndrome. In: *Surgery of the Musculoskeletal System,* CMcC Evarts, ed. New York: Churchill-Livingstone, 1983.
12. Evarts CMcC and Mayer PJ. Complications: The fat embolism syndrome. In: *Fractures in Adults: Volume 1,* 2nd edition. Rockwood CA Jr, Green DP, eds. Philadelphia: J. B. Lippincott, 1984.
13. Fess EE, Philips CA. *Hand Splinting: Principles and Methods.* St. Louis: C. V. Mosby, 1987.
14. Goldman L. Cardiac risks and complications of noncardiac surgery. **Annals of Surgery,** 198(6): 780-791, 1983.
15. Goldman L, Caldera DL, Nussbaum SR et al. Multifactorial index of cardiac risk in noncardiac surgical procedures. **N. Engl. J. Med.,** 297: 845, 1977.
16. Hughes M, Neer CS. Glenohumeral joint replacement and postoperative rehabilitation. **Physical Therapy,** 55: 850, 1975.
17. Hull RD, Raskob GE, Hirsh J. Prophylaxis of venous thromboembolism. **Chest,** 89(5) [Supplement]: 374S-382S, 1986.
18. Kortz WJ, Lumb PD, eds. *Surgical Intensive Care: A Practical Guide.* Chicago: Yearbook Medical Publishers, 1984.
19. Lowe LW. Venous thrombosis and embolism. **JBJS-B,** 63B(2): 155-167, 1981.

20. Mubarak SJ. Compartment syndromes. In: MW Chapman, ed. *Operative Orthopaedics*. Philadelphia: J. B. Lippincott, 1988.

21. Ranamurthy S. Anesthesia. In: Green DP, ed. *Operative Hand Surgery*. 1st edition. New York: Churchill Livingstone, 1982.

22. Redford JB. *Orthotics Etcetera*. 3rd edition. Baltimore: Williams & Wilkins, 1986.

23. Sabiston DC Jr. "Pulmonary embolism" In: Sabiston DC Jr, ed. *Textbook of Surgery: The Biological Basis of Modern Surgical Practice*. 13th edition. Philadelphia: W. B. Saunders, 1986.

24. Schirmer BD, Sabiston DC Jr. "Preoperative preparation of the surgical patient." In: Sabiston DC Jr, ed. *Essentials of Surgery*. Philadelphia: W. B. Saunders, 1987.

25. Teitz CC et al. Evaluation of the use of braces to prevent injury in collegiate football players. **JBJS**, 69A: 2, 1987.

26. Tisi GM. Preoperative evaluation of pulmonary function: validity, indications, and benefits. **American Review of Respiratory Disease, 119**: 293-309, 1979.

27. Zarins B, Rowe CR. Combined anterior cruciate ligament reconstruction using semitendinosus tendon and iliotibial tract. **JBJS**, 68A: 160, 1986.

Index

Page numbers in *italics* denote figures